RECALCULATING

Travels Along the Road Through Crisis

Amy Dempsey

iUniverse, Inc.
Bloomington

RECALCULATING
Travels Along the Road Through Crisis

iUniverse books may be ordered through booksellers or by contacting:

iUniverse
1663 Liberty Drive
Bloomington, IN 47403
www.iuniverse.com
1-800-Authors (1-800-288-4677)

ISBN: 978-1-4759-3874-6 (sc)
ISBN: 978-1-4759-3876-0 (hc)
ISBN: 978-1-4759-3875-3 (ebk)

Printed in the United States of America

iUniverse rev. date: 07/27/2012

For Garry Burros, who brought out the best in everyone

Introduction

I lost my job in February of 2009 and soon after that shoe dropped I found out that I had breast cancer. After months of making difficult decisions and choices regarding my health, a diversion was badly needed. If I could have reinvented myself that would have been beneficial. Unfortunately, there were no ideas and so I stuck to recuperating. I began to keep a journal and found this endeavor more enjoyable than any job I ever received payment for.

During my recovery, my attention and focus were altered drastically when my brother Garry was diagnosed with amyotrophic lateral sclerosis or ALS, which is often referred to as Lou Gehrig's disease. I quickly found that having to focus on more than one or two major issues at once was merely a fact of life. People offered their interest and concern in different ways. All their efforts brought great comfort. Being able to extend some support in return, when it was needed by them, was equally rewarding for me.

Because I believe that life is about what we share and not about what we face, I have decided to do just that. Admittedly I am an ordinary woman. I am not a hero, an intellectual, a successful entrepreneur, a celebrity, or anyone else of any real stature. Most of us are ordinary people with unique and interesting lives. Add the perspective gained through crisis and the lessons are invaluable.

This two-year period in my life reveals the complexity of emotions in managing medical crisis, placing a loved one in a nursing home, coping with grief and other family issues. Though I often doubted my ability to navigate through the detours that came along, I found it was easier to find my way with help. The best thing, of course, is to have a good support system and I was very fortunate in that regard.

Breast cancer brought me a huge challenge that started me on a journey to prove difficult situations can be managed, while moving forward at the same time. What I soon discovered was strength found in relationships all around, which brought me the resolution I needed to keep going.

Being somewhat of a fraidy-cat, a negative person and a worrier it was not always easy for me to appreciate many of the positive things that were also happening. Important and good times could have been easily diminished by what we were all going through, but I chose not to let that happen. That determination allowed me to fully enjoy our daughter's high school play performance, despite my brother's grave condition and other concerns. I was touched by the many contrasts life frequently presented, allowing me to be filled with sorrow and joy often simultaneously.

Months into my breast cancer experience I decided to keep a journal to record my experiences and emotions. Entries based on a medical diary I kept separately were easily included to accurately tell how this all began. At times I wrote daily, but often I would use chronological notes jotted down in between to catch up on longer periods of time.

Remaining involved in daily events brought a better balance to circumstances that often overwhelmed and tested me. The entire writing process helped me to evaluate everything in a more positive way, easing much of the pain and fear of both mine and my brother's crises.

Describing Garry was a way of preserving a bit of the extraordinary and rare person that he was. My brother had faced mental retardation, cerebral palsy and a cleft palate since birth. He was a self-sufficient member of a group home and held a twenty-eight year job that was a great source of pride for him. He became a role model and an advocate for the mentally challenged. Garry led his life with dignity and kindness and was beloved by all who were fortunate to know him. It was a privilege for me to describe him and tell of his plight with the devastating disease which robbed him of everything he had, except the love he had deservedly earned.

The details I have chosen to include offer an intimate view of a family handling all the issues that go on through these times. For me, remaining "present" to the best of my ability was essential to my recovery and sanity. Documenting this period lets me clearly remember the lessons I experienced firsthand, which human nature and time often alter and reconstruct. The omission of any names, events, or kindnesses are not a reflection of their importance, but done to simplify telling about these two years.

Finally, I realized how much faith I had. That was not a small task for this glass-half-empty gal. My fondest hope is that this memoir will bring some comfort and inspiration to others, like myself, who sometimes doubt they will find their way.

B.B.C.
(BEFORE BREAST CANCER)

At age fifty I found my way back to working outside my home. Being a person who was sorely lacking in any marketable skills, this was not easy. I began with a job in daycare and soon decided that this was not a good fit. Then I tried telemarketing which was just awful. Finally, I worked in customer service at a small educational equipment company for about three years. When the economy changed, I was let go. Although it was a relatively unimportant position, it was still humiliating when it happened.

After joining the ranks of the unemployed I decided to make some positive changes. I wanted to get back to a walking program which I had done before returning to work outside my home six years before. This also seemed like the ideal time to get some medical appointments taken care of as I had a variety of concerns. Juggling my part-time job, a family of five and the responsibilities of a household, things were often set aside for later. It was time to regain better control and make improvements.

A friend from high school was out of work, also. Ginny and I found walking for exercise essential to dealing with our situations, and did our best to get into a routine. Her husband was also a former classmate and friend of ours. My husband John and I always get an enormous kick out of this couple. Due to our circumstances Ginny and I were becoming closer than ever. Both of us were feeling unsettled and it helped to have someone else who really understood to talk with. Unlike myself, my friend is highly qualified in her field. We were both faced with the dilemma of finding a new job at our ages in this bleak economy.

My sister Vicki and I also began meeting to walk regularly. This was particularly good for our relationship. It allowed us to spend more time together and rediscover the closeness that we had previously enjoyed. As I had been lost in Mommydom, while she was equally submerged in running her own successful real estate business, it was sometimes difficult for us to stay connected.

Some mornings Ginny, Vicki and I walked together. Vicki's daughter Jennifer is a strikingly fit, thirty-something woman living on her own in Manhattan; occasionally she would stay over in New Jersey and join us. It was pleasant time spent doing something we were sure was good for us all, and the mental health boost of their friendship was welcomed.

Women need to talk about their experiences. They have to vent and laugh whenever possible with someone who "gets-it." Men, and this is not judgmental, need sex, or some form of competition or hobby to help keep them going. None of these actions provide all the answers to life's challenges. They do, in my opinion, often make things a little easier and more tolerable.

By now it was May of 2009. I was fifty-six and due for my routine annual mammography. As always, there was some anxiety involved.

My family has a very strong history of breast cancer. My mom's sister was diagnosed more than forty years ago and had a mastectomy; today she is in her eighties. My dad was diagnosed with breast cancer at age fifty-six and had a mastectomy. This was the first time I realized that this disease also affected men. Sadly, he passed away at fifty-eight in 1983. Several years later, my sister Vicki was diagnosed at thirty-eight with the same disease and also had a mastectomy.

From the beginning Vicki became proactive and rededicated herself to "living." She learned to eliminate certain stresses, and became a more positive person. My sister identified the things that brought her the most purpose and enjoyment in her life and concentrated on them. From the time Vicki was first diagnosed I started to go for annual screenings.

This year I was aware of more breast pain than usual, so I was perhaps a bit more concerned about my test. My highly cystic breasts always presented difficulty in proper imaging. Routinely there would be two to four sets of images taken before I would be allowed to leave the breast center.

During the screening the technician explained that the new digital camera required a particularly compressed position to obtain maximum results. It shocked me to see my breasts reduced to flat pancakes and as became very uncomfortable, I complained. The mammography was performed on May 15, 2009. From that time on, I attributed the stronger pain in my breasts, especially on my left side, and pain in my ribs to that test. This discomfort stayed with me for months.

The breast center notified me that a breast MRI was appropriate. They stated the request was based on family history. It had been a number of years since I had taken this test. With the amount of pain I was experiencing this was easily agreed to.

June came and I had the MRI. I was nervous. My doctor notified me that an area on my right breast needed more imaging, an ultrasound and a possible needle biopsy. This was not surprising. I still thought that something was up with my left breast as there was substantially more discomfort on that side.

I went to this appointment by myself as usual. I never thought it necessary to have company for any of these tests and these places are always overcrowded anyway. I went from additional mammography to having an ultrasound.

The doctor had taken time and great care in locating and examining the area. I sensed her discovery and some concern, which I felt she was silently showing her assistant. I asked, "Do you have a conclusion you can share with me?" She stopped, looked deep into my eyes and replied, "Are you the kind of person who really wants to hear that answer? Or are you the kind who needs to have the official report after the pathology comes back?" I said, "I want to hear it right now, from you."

The doctor carefully explained her conclusion as she retraced what she was looking at on the monitor. She was certain that this was a small cancerous tumor. Her honesty and clinical manner was appreciated. Next, she performed one core biopsy and two fine-needle biopsies.

I moved and got nicked accidentally with the needle used to do the biopsy and I began to bleed. At this point I started to cry; not the sobbing kind, just the quiet, streaming variety. The nurses and doctor were supportive and caring. I quickly composed myself. One more imaging was required to make sure the clip left during the core biopsy was in its correct place for the future procedure required.

I left thinking, *Finally the thing I was prepared to hear for years has happened.*

Three days later when my general practitioner called to say he received the report, it was still shocking as he explained, "Amy, it is bad news. You will have to see a breast surgeon as soon as possible." He never said "cancer." My doctor simply sounded emphatic and alarmed.

I got off the phone and found my husband. Though John and I had discussed what happened at my appointment days earlier, this call came as a second blow. After quickly hugging one another, we thought of our three children who were all home. Instinctively we had to collect ourselves.

John and I saw no need to share the news yet. We all had planned to see the fireworks display on July 3, in the next town. Sitting through the noisy celebration, I can remember feeling like I wasn't really there.

I do recall John saying before we went to sleep, "Look, if they suggest a mastectomy, you might want to consider having both breasts done." I took that as a sign that he could handle his end of this situation.

So, this is where my breast cancer journey really begins.

STARTING MY JOURNEY

My husband and I hosted a Fourth of July family BBQ, where we successfully avoided telling our family about my situation. That felt right because we hadn't gotten any medical advice and we were uncertain what course would be taken. We pulled off the summer celebration with no one suspecting that anything was wrong.

However, I did end up confiding in John's sister Mary after everyone else went home. We have been quite close and shared many issues over the years. I knew she could be counted on to help my family out, if needed.

Telling my mother and sister would be more difficult; I knew how worried they would become. My walking pal Ginny knew about my screening and tests from the get-go. This made it easier to tell her about the breast cancer diagnosis. I told her right away, of course, she was totally supportive. One thing I discovered each time I told someone: it made it easier to tell the next one. I waited to share my crisis with a couple of other friends until after I shared the "news" with my family.

Sunday, John and I sat our children down, and let them know what was going on. It was summer time. I knew they would be around overhearing all kinds of phone conversations between me and doctors' offices and our insurance company. Anne was twenty-four; Keith was twenty and Cara was almost fifteen years old. They were not babies. It seemed wise to be open and honest from the beginning. They were concerned, but they also seemed confident that we would do whatever was needed to be done.

Later that evening I told my sister, who was a twenty-three year breast cancer survivor; she was surprisingly calm, and assured me she would help me. Vicki can be a tower of strength, but *she* must be in control. She is the biggest advocate of the power of positive thinking outside of Oprah. I am sure she was distraught, but I did not detect that at all. We agreed my mother and my step-dad, Irwin, should be told later on when I had more information.

Mom married Irwin about six years after my dad passed away. Irwin's son (from another marriage) and his family live in Colorado. Mom and Irwin were expecting his son Alan and two of their grandsons for a special visit. Irwin, my husband John and our son Keith joined the three of them to see a baseball game at the new Yankee Stadium. We saw no reason to put a blemish on this time by telling about my diagnosis, yet. That was definitely the right move as everyone had a great weekend.

In the meantime, I tried to find a surgeon. This brought me to a specialist in a nearby hospital. I scheduled an appointment with the doctor after she returned from her vacation two weeks later.

July 20, 2009, was my first consultation with a breast surgeon. My sister Vicki and John went with me. I was fully prepared with films, a CD, reports, and my plastic file folder chock-full of all my medical information gathered from the past year. I had created my own records of my other medical concerns, symptoms and history. It may seem unnecessary; however, this system has come in handy on a number of appointments.

The doctor was a foreign-born woman who exuded strength and firmness. She evaluated my records and family history. Quickly, she expressed her recommendation for a mastectomy. The explanation included: her hand-drawn diagrams of the breast, key information, and success rates of the various options. The doctor said, "Your tumor is an early-stage, slow-growing and garden-variety breast cancer."

It was hearing her say I had breast cancer while looking into my eyes, as she explained the situation and options, which made it finally sink in. Before this, I thought, *"I got it."* Nope. There must have been some doubt or denial in my mind. How crazy! This doctor cleared that right up. Unconsciously, I hoped a misunderstanding or an error had occurred. Honestly, I did not even realize I felt that way.

The doctor insisted on me taking the hereditary gene test for breast and ovarian cancer right there and then. It is called the BRCA test. She felt certain the results would make my decision clearer. Those results would take about two weeks to get back. Sending me for a chest x-ray also, I knew she was thinking about surgery—soon. The tests were done there that same day.

I told this doctor I had an appointment for a second opinion. She appeared momentarily "put-off," but asked me to let her know of my decision. I am very grateful for her directness, her insistence that I needed the gene test results, and her assurance that we were dealing with this at an early and manageable time.

My second appointment three days later was with my sister's surgeon. This appointment was at a prominent and well-respected hospital. It made sense to me to get a second opinion where they have the best, updated equipment and the most experienced specialists.

My sister had asked her breast doctor's office for a suitable referral for me, thinking my insurance company was not in-network with their hospital. The doctor's nurse told her that they were just becoming affiliated with my insurance company. Vicki called me in tears. She was so happy that I could go to this hospital without additional issues. It struck both of us that this was a divine intervention.

Vicki has long credited her breast cancer survival to this hospital and her original doctor, who was killed in an accident about six years ago. She was a brilliant surgeon and researcher considered to be tops in her field; her loss is still acknowledged throughout the hospital.

John and Vicki accompanied me again on this second consultation. The second doctor was a young, soft-spoken woman. She avoided telling me what to do and preferred to go over the facts and details of my situation. The statistics were an important part of the consultation as well. It seemed confusing as it all boiled down to the fact: *Survival is equal—with a mastectomy or a lumpectomy.*

The lumpectomy offered breast conservation. It was to be followed by seven weeks of radiation therapy and routine six-month checkups. This plan included mammography and MRI tests alternating for years to come. The breast surgeon said, "In your particular case with this tumor, the decision is one only you can make." She added, "If the situation was different I might feel more inclined to guide you more in a particular direction." There was so much to think over. We also wanted to have the results from the BRCA test, as the statistics were greatly affected by the hereditary gene.

About a week later, the first surgeon called me with the results from the test. I was positive for the BRCA 2 gene. We spoke about the second consult. This doctor made it clear that the test results had taken away the lumpectomy option. I appreciated her advice, but I preferred to go with the New York hospital. Our conversation was brief, and she wished me well.

The decision had to be right for me. Of course, my decision would also be important to those I love as well.

At first, I thought the lumpectomy made good sense. It would be less drastic and definitely easier on my body with less recovery. There would be one operation vs. the more substantial mastectomy surgery and reconstruction, which requires two operations in my case. After a few days passed, I realized my heart was telling me to think more about the mastectomy. Reducing the chances of reoccurrences was a big deal to me.

Realizing that the risks of recurrences were higher with lumpectomy just did not sit well with me. I recalled years before when I was going for a mammography and breast MRIs at six-month intervals to watch an area of concern. That constant testing made me anxious and uncomfortable. It felt as though I was on "cancer alert" which drove me a little crazy. After obtaining a second opinion I switched my routine diagnostics to a different facility where it was a little less intense.

Recalling the earlier experiences, I had to ask myself if *I* could handle the constant testing, and the watch-and-find course that lumpectomy offered. Surely some people would find this preferable to mastectomy. Would it be best for me? Would it be best for my family? Either way there was "no one hundred percent guarantee" that this breast cancer would not return. Finally, my decision became clear. I called the surgeon's office and told them I had decided on a double mastectomy. They told me to come in for another consultation.

Again, we all went to the doctor's office where I explained how I came to the decision. The general consensus was that the pain in my left breast was not of concern at this time—I was still somewhat unconvinced. My preference was to do both breasts at one time. It eliminated the worry of cancer returning in the other breast someday. My body would be the same on both sides, which made better sense to me.

The surgeon appeared to be fine with my decision. She explained, "Patients, in my experience, are most comfortable coming to their own decisions, as opposed to being talked into something." Lastly, we talked about scheduling an operation.

The doctor felt strongly that I needed to see a gynecological surgeon to talk about an oophorectomy, the removal of the ovaries and tubes. This would eliminate the estrogen produced by the ovaries, might increase chances of breast cancer returning. The BRCA 2 gene puts me at greater risk to develop ovarian cancer, too. As there is currently no good diagnostics for detecting early-stage ovarian cancer, this needed to be considered as well. Wow! This was more than I expected to have to think about. In addition, we needed to see a plastic surgeon about reconstruction. Jeepers, what the heck? Appointments to see these other doctors for consultations were set up immediately.

Most people seemed relieved that I chose to get the mastectomy done. I felt support all around me. John had been very careful not to try and influence me in any way. He and I think very differently in the area of medical attention. John has had a handful of personal experiences that has made him skeptical and mistrustful. My husband does not like being rushed to make any decision, and really dislikes not being in complete control. He was less convinced.

I was looking to put myself in "good hands" and wanted to weigh my options and make informed decisions. I believed that divine intervention had been in play already; my faith was strong that I would become a breast cancer survivor.

On August 3 I went for my consultation with the gynecologist. My husband and sister came with me. The doctor was a tall, handsome man, who had an air of warmth about him. He spoke unwaveringly about removing the ovaries. He explained, "The ovaries provide less that is good at this point, and the benefit from removal is much greater. The ovaries and tubes are removed and the uterus is checked out. Remember, as you head toward seventy years old your chances are substantially increased for ovarian cancer with the BRCA gene. The fact that you are post-menopausal is actually an advantage."

The gynecologist recommended this additional procedure be done during the second operation, when the permanent implants are put in by the plastic surgeon. Since I would be under anesthesia anyway, this meant one less operation another time. What a deal, two operations and one anesthesia in one day! We all agreed that this would be done. The gynecologist was personable and very persuasive.

The next day the meeting with the plastic surgeon was informative. He was slight of build and extremely serious in manner. Both the plastic surgeon and the gynecologist were very specialized and instilled confidence in different ways. The plastic surgeon was direct and armed with details.

John, Vicki and I had no idea how complicated reconstruction is. The plastic surgeon explained different options; none were a single step. He said, "Women your age should have the reconstruction done; however, you will never like the implants as much as your natural breasts. I want to give women their best option after breast cancer surgery." There were many pictures to look at and samples of implants and lots of information. Our heads were exploding! In my case, implants seemed to be the best choice. I had a choice from three different kinds; two were filled with silicone material and one with saline and all had silicone outer material. I had more time to make this decision.

The doctor told us that he would come in after the mastectomy was done, and place the tissue expanders under the muscles in my chest. They would fill these slightly at that time. There would be four or five subsequent office visits to fill them with a little more fluid each time. The doctor noted that he planned to reduce the size of my breasts. You look for some "good" anywhere you can find it in these situations. This was probably the closest thing I had heard for a while. The reconstruction would stretch out the whole process for another four months or more. This plastic surgeon had an excellent reputation, and I was certain that I would have him do my reconstruction.

There was one more issue. At the time of the mastectomy, the lymph nodes are checked for any cancer involvement. This determines whether removal is required and if so, chemotherapy prescribed. If the lymph nodes are clear, which is good then, the tumor is still tested. This test evaluates how effective chemotherapy is on this particular tumor. Should the score from the test indicate enough benefit, chemo would be recommended. We were not talking about future new cancers; we were still talking about the recurrence of this same breast cancer. I couldn't believe it!

If any stray cancer cell(s) remain behind an active cancer could develop again. Chemotherapy would target and kill any dividing breast cancer cells. There are patients that are saved by having this therapy. This is sort of an insurance plan. All of the information and decisions blew my mind! I felt in charge and out of control at the same time.

Sharing the News

Knowing what my options were, I decided to let Mom and Irwin in on what was going on. I was concerned about them because there already was a lot on their plate. My mom's brother-in-law Leon had fallen and he was hospitalized with bleeding on his brain. Mom and Irwin were running back and forth to help my mom's sister Betty and to see him. This had gone on for several weeks.

In addition, my brother Garry was having serious medical problems that had become obvious over the past year. Having been born intellectually challenged, and with cerebral palsy, it appeared that the CP had now reared its ugly head, creating new and more difficult issues. Garry had lost the use of both legs and his left arm and hand. The doctors were not quite sure what was going on yet. This was a shocking change that had taken place over a period of six to eight months. First he managed with a walker. Soon that became impossible for him and he needed to be in a wheelchair. Add my situation to the pile and it was already a terrible time for our family.

With the wisdom of older people, who have seen many problems come and go, Mom and Irwin were not letting my news throw them. Listening to me carefully they finally said, "Amy, we know you will make the right decisions about how to handle this."

I expected my mom to get very upset, and this was such a relief. I turned to Irwin and said, "*You*, you went to the new Yankee Stadium last weekend and cried. My news doesn't bring a tear?" I admit now it was a bad joke. He started to cry, "Amy, if you knew how I feel about you." I quickly apologized and said, "I know." Admittedly I felt a little comfort in this display of emotion. Letting them know what was going on was an enormous load off my mind.

My surgery was scheduled for August 14, 2009. The breast surgeon would perform the double mastectomy and then, the plastic surgeon would start the reconstruction immediately. It was coming up fast.

The next person I wanted to tell was my close friend Laura. We have shared so much since meeting in junior high school. Her response kind of surprised me: "Oh Amy, I am so sorry. I don't know what to say, I am sure you'll be OK." She was obviously upset and thrown by my news, and I detected a little fright in her trembling voice. I knew that once she got past the shock that I could count on her support.

I also confided in my neighbor Dee. She is a sweetheart of a gal, who faced breast cancer years ago. She opted for a different reconstruction, where no implant is used. Instead, they put your own tissue from another area, often from the stomach, and fill in the removed breast tissue. It is a delicate and lengthy surgery. It has its advantages and yet there are risks specific to this surgery. Dee was open and helpful; hers was a spontaneous cancer. Like my sister, my neighbor also has a tremendously positive attitude. Being around people like them is incredibly helpful.

Naming all the loved ones, friends, or supportive acquaintances that have extended themselves to me would be impossible. It is indescribable how moving it is to receive the kindnesses of others. At this point, sharing my crisis with people seemed like a way of gathering their prayers, good wishes and positive energy.

John contacted an old high school friend who moved to North Carolina years ago. We saw Carol and her husband at one or two reunions. We also saw them a few years ago when she came back to New Jersey for a memorial service for her younger sister, who had passed away from breast cancer. Carol has breast cancer, too. She had been keeping us updated through e-mail on her latest cancer reoccurrence. Knowing she was having a tough time with her chemotherapy, we were very concerned about her. Now Carol was keeping my spirits up by sending me cards and notes. Her encouragements are particularly meaningful.

My sister Vicki has been my rock throughout this experience, literally putting her business on hold for every appointment I have. I know that even thinking of going in and out of New York would be nearly impossible for me if it were not for her. Sure, John could do some of that; however, it would be a real infringement on his office time. My sister's schedule is much more flexible and so far it has been working.

I don't drive in the city. I don't know my way around and frankly, driving there is far too aggressive for me. Vicki is convinced I don't even walk around the city well. It is true that with all the trips we have made already, I never seem to remember which direction we need to go in. Vicki, on the other hand, is a city-girl and feels at home whenever we are in New York. So far this all seems to be workable.

On the weekend before my surgery, John and I went out to dinner with his sister Mary and her husband Bob. John made a surprising disclosure. He confided in them that he had finally told me that he would choose the lumpectomy surgery *this* time. They were somewhat taken aback. Mary told John, "When Amy called me with her decision to have a mastectomy instead of a lumpectomy; I started to cry because I was so relieved."

John respected my right to have the final decision. Yet, he needed to go on record that he felt a lumpectomy might be sufficient adding, "If there are any recurrences—absolutely, go ahead with a mastectomy then." It hurt me a little, but he was honest and afraid and I understood. After that conversation he continued to be only supportive.

We were busy with all kinds of details and arrangements for the next week. In the midst of everything that was going on, my feisty Uncle Leon passed away. His immediate family respected his wishes to be cremated. My aunt and cousins decided to delay the memorial service until two weeks after my surgery. This allowed me an opportunity to attend if, I was able to. It also gave me my first goal of sorts.

Oddly enough, Leon was going to do one more thing just for me. I have to jump ahead a few days here. The night before my surgery I started to doze off in front of the TV. I awoke in a short time startled. I had seen a man walking down an empty, brightly lit hallway toward me. I finally recognized a younger Leon wearing a white t-shirt, plaid shorts, light blue socks and white sneakers. He had a peaceful expression—not happy or sad. I remember thinking, *My God; he's coming to take me with him!*

After a moment, I realized he was telling me that I would be OK. It was a dream, of course. Was it more? I don't know for sure, but it brought me a sense of extra protection. Thanks, Uncle Lee!

—m—

The week of my mastectomy Vicki and I had to go into New York three times for appointments. There were doctor appointments with details to go over and pre-surgery tests to be done. Testing put me in waiting areas with many patients with all kinds of cancer. The saddest thing is seeing the young children who are there. That offered me perspective on how fortunate I was.

The whole week felt a little surreal. My operation was scheduled for August 14, 2009, at 12:30. I was to be admitted at 10:30 in the morning. Thank God, John and Vicki were able to accompany me. Knowing neither of them would be alone was also comforting for me. Truth be told, my idea of surgery is having my ears pierced and I was very nervous. However, after waiting for six weeks to deal with this cancer, I just wanted it to be over.

My main priority was to show my children that life's emergencies can be handled. Falling apart or feeling sorry for me, was not what I wanted them to see. I needed them to know I had the strength and conviction to deal with whatever needed to be done. This was very important to me.

After dinner the night before the surgery, our daughters insisted that we have a combination good luck and anniversary celebration. Our son Keith was unfortunately at work so he was missing. They had cards for us and a delicious ice-cream cake. The three kids had gone to the park earlier that day and taken some photos. They each wore a light-pink t-shirt and held a one word sign: WE—LOVE—YOU, all written in bubble letters. A friend helped to take the pictures. They thought that I would want to take one with me to the hospital.

I was very happy that they had thought of such a sweet thing to do. They even had one picture turned into a puzzle for me to work on. The doctor had said after my operation I might have a slight manual dexterity issue. They thought a puzzle would be somewhat therapeutic and helpful.

John and I were going to be married thirty-four years on that Sunday; the same day I would come home from the hospital. The girls wisely thought that it might not be the easiest day to plan any kind of celebration. Seeing how my family was handling everything thus far was very reassuring.

Mom and Irwin stopped by to wish me luck and said they could be called if any help would be needed in the weeks ahead. I could tell Mom had it under control. I noticed she had added a second breast cancer pin near the collar of her blouse which stood for both of her daughters. Only Ms. Accessory herself could think to make this statement, this way.

In trying to be thorough, I reinstructed my family on how to run the dishwasher and the laundry machines. I offered them all sorts of reminders about lights, locks, driving and more. Oh boy, now I was in a panic! I even left a stack of index cards with the same information on the kitchen table. Included with those was the list of phone numbers of people who asked to be called after the operation. This was all the information they needed to know if something went terribly wrong.

We were all set. I had prepared meals ahead of time and left them in the freezer to make the week after surgery easier on us all. In my mind I could be gone for two days or maybe forever. I was trying to be strong; actually, I was scared to my core.

SURGERY

Vicki drove the three of us into the city the morning of August 14, 2009. John jokingly wondered aloud if he should be insulted this was an implication he might not be up to that job. We both knew it made my sister more comfortable and we remained calm.

We arrived early and went through the usual process of admission. Eventually, we found ourselves seated in a large waiting area. As you looked around you became more familiar with that somber expression that almost everyone wore. Patients and companions alike seemed ready to go through the motions, and prepared to camp out waiting for their chance to "make things better."

Vicki, John and I made a little small talk and just waited to hear my name called. After some time, we were moved to another area where I was given a hospital gown and my IV. Then, the wait really began.

My scheduled surgery was running quite late. Every so often we were directed to a different location. Finally a nurse parked us in a small space close to the operating room where it felt like we spent forever. My surgery was close to three hours late when it was my turn. It was a long day without eating. After a while you can get a bit delirious and there were even moments of humor. I supplied my companions with lollipops toward the end of this time. My husband and sister wished me luck. I was sure we were all silently saying, *Thank God, it's about time!*

A young nurse called me to follow her and asked me to identify myself with my name and birth date. As we started to walk off she asked me where I lived. When I told her, she became very interested. She had lived nearby and was familiar with the area. We walked toward the operating room as though we were friends going to get a cup of coffee together.

The anesthesiologist introduced herself to me next. Then, I saw my surgeon and I remember her stroking my arm. We spoke only seconds before I was unconscious.

Later I remember waking only briefly to see John and Vicki standing near my bed. They reassured me that everything went fine. The nurses told them I would sleep most of the rest of the night. I could see a balloon at the foot of the bed left by my niece Jennifer, who had come by earlier. I vaguely recall being concerned about whether my husband and sister had eaten anything. Then I thought, *Those two definitely took care of that—they surely needed and deserved a good meal and a stiff drink today.* They told me they were leaving to go home and I slipped back to sleep.

Sometime in the middle of the night I woke up. It was shockingly impossible to navigate off my bed. I was in pain, unsteady and nauseous. The nurse came and helped me manage to get out of bed and back again. She explained, "The pain medication is delivered in the IV at the push of a button, and it will *not* allow you to over medicate." She recommended strongly, "Take it as often as needed." Normally, I even resist aspirin. However, now this system was appealing and seemed to be a rather splendid idea!

The next morning I felt as if a bus hit me. I became nauseous every time I got out of bed. Before long, I received instructions about taking care of myself at home the next day. Yikes! Feeling the way I did—they were kidding, right?

I introduced myself to my roommate Donna. She had ovarian cancer. This was her third hospitalization since her diagnosis. Once in a while you meet a person who you know has an amazing spirit, and she was one of them. What impressed me most about Donna was the way she treated everyone she spoke with. My roommate greeted every nurse, doctor, and phone caller with optimism, grace and humor. She wore her brightly-colored head scarves confidently and with great flair.

We chatted, and I felt guilty to complain about how I was feeling this morning. Yet, it was difficult not to say anything about that either. She was very understanding. I hoped that I could be half as strong as she seemed to be.

John came back in the morning and I was glad to see him. He said the kids were thinking they wanted to come, too. We had both discouraged that idea. I knew that my hospital stay was brief, and that this would likely be a tough day.

I needed instructions on the at-home care of my drains, and that alone made me a bit anxious. The surgeon had placed two drains at each side of my chest, below my armpits. It was odd to see the four bulbs, and the tubes that came from them leading into my body. These let the extra fluid, which is produced from the surgery and healing process, leave your body to help avoid infection. The bulbs had to be emptied two times each day after surgery, and until your body produced less than a certain amount in a day. That was to take a week to ten days. I wanted to be sure I could take care of myself post-surgery. John and I agreed that it was going to be a challenging day and our children need not be in on this.

It all worked out well. Grandma and Grandpa had taken their grandkids out to breakfast. That is my mom's favorite medicine for all situations and it works pretty well most of the time.

Later on Aunt Mary and Uncle Bob took Anne and Cara to see their cousin in a summer school musical production. Both girls thought Dan was absolutely great in his role. So, their day was pretty special. Keith had other plans which he did not change. All was good. We knew we had made the right decision.

To get back to my one full day in the hospital recovering from surgery: One very sweet young nurse came in to talk with us. She wanted to go over taking care of the drains at home. She also explained, "You must take a good look at the incisions, and get familiar with what is normal looking just in case any changes occur." She asked, "Are you OK with John looking also?" We both agreed. Honestly, I was pretty scared as I am terribly squeamish. She handed me a large mirror while John stood still in his place. The nurse's demeanor was gentle and kind. I felt her compassion and concern, for both of us. She took off the bandages and assured us everything looked as it should.

John was great. Whatever he was thinking, I never felt that he was shocked, repulsed or even upset. He was very strong. It was important that this had taken place right there and then.

Looking in that mirror for the first time was a very sad moment for me. *This was the result of a choice I had made. I was changed forever.*

The incisions looked weird, the expanders were evident, and my coloring a little strange. The drains added to my bizarre appearance. I took a good look; and *that* moment was over. John was particularly wonderful.

We sat together afterward and made small talk, while watching some TV, but my nausea kept getting worse.

My breast surgeon stopped in to examine me before she left for a week of vacation. She looked casual in her breast-cancer-pink button down shirt, over a tank-shirt, white cropped pants and sandals. Looking beautiful, and at least five years younger than I remembered her looking in her doctor's garb, she told me, "Everything went well." I mentioned the nausea and she immediately ordered some medication, which I gladly ingested.

John and I decided to go for a walk. Within minutes we had to rush back to my room. John quickly put a waste basket up to my face in a quick decision to allow me to throw up. I must have gotten sick four or more times violently. Afterward, I felt a thousand percent better. I ordered a meal right away and was glad when it arrived.

Donna's husband came in to our room and we all sat together for quite a while. We were four good people just trying to do our best to get through an awful time. They were easy to talk with and very interesting. Her husband had been an officer in the Armed Forces until finally the Middle East situation forced him in "good conscience" to resign. She had been a successful professional before she became a soldier in her own war against cancer. They had a family they obviously adored. Donna was having her best day, and was determined to leave on the next. I was rather apprehensive about being dismissed. She was already a veteran at this hospital stuff. I was obviously recently drafted.

John and I did lots of hall walking that day. I was actually doing quite well with that. My exercising these past months helped. We walked, talked, and watched some TV for the remainder of that day. Every so often, someone would stop by to check on me, but mostly we were left on our own.

Sometime in the afternoon, we noticed that my coloring had turned deep-red especially on my chest, neck and face. My chest and shoulders were starting to appear almost purple. The nurse realized I was having a reaction to some medication. I had noticed some chest tightness earlier, and was confused by what I thought were issues from the surgery. The doctor immediately switched the antibiotic and administered allergy medication. I was back to my normal color again and feeling fine in a short time. John left later in the evening.

The covering plastic surgeon came by that night to examine me and remarked, "This was a relatively minor surgery." To which he must have seen the lack of agreement on my face and said, "You know, this is a surgery on the outside as opposed to one on the inside of your body." He was cold in his bedside manner, and I was annoyed with him. I knew then, I was ready to go home.

The morning of August 16 things went quickly. I was a sight in my huge shirt, which failed to hide the four bulbs underneath. I left the hospital carefully. My roommate and I swapped personal information; we were both eager to leave. I brought a pillow from home for protection in the car in case of short stops or bumps. It was a relief that this surgery was behind me and I was glad to go home. Neither John nor I gave our anniversary any thought.

My sister and her husband Paul picked us up from the hospital and drove us home. I remember how strong he had been about handling Vicki's breast cancer crisis years earlier. John and I were so grateful to have their support now.

Our brother-in-law Bob had dropped off a large foam-rubber wedge for under my bed pillows, which was extremely helpful. Other than that, there were not many differences. We had discussed some additional duties for our children. I could not lift much, and they were going to assist around the house more than usual. John returned to work on Monday knowing I had lots of help. It was still summer and our children would be at home.

Recovery Begins

Anne was thoughtful, and had taken this first week as some of her vacation time from her work at the bank. Normally, that would seem silly to me. As far as I knew, she neither cooked nor cleaned much of anything. Let me say for the record, Anne was great. She did her best to do as much as possible. I cannot imagine how I would have managed without her.

Cara too, was pitching in. She became the laundry maven. She and John did most of the vacuuming in the first couple of weeks. Our children were handling things well and that was gratifying to me. John returned to work knowing things were in good hands.

Keith had been reserved about my cancer. He simply told me, "Mom you're strong and I am sure you'll be fine." I felt his sincerity and his love. Communication has never been his favorite sport, but he seemed OK with all this. His main duty was to get ready to go back to school.

It was his junior year at Rutgers University. Normally we had worked together getting him ready. I was disappointed about not helping Keith move into his apartment this year missing the opportunity to meet all his new roommates. Anne volunteered to do this big job. The two of them felt that everything was well under control and I knew they were right. John was exhausted and appreciated Anne's help here. She was a life saver for us all; the weekend after my surgery Keith was off to college.

We received many food contributions from various family and friends, which were both a help and a treat. There were flowers, fruit baskets, cards, lots of goodies and thoughtful good wishes delivered over the next weeks. I felt very loved and supported. I gave "thanks" for every gesture and good thought—it was an overwhelming experience. You cannot believe how kind people can be; and *not* just the people you always count on, or those who are expected to be concerned.

I went for about nine days with the drains and it was great to get rid of them! While waiting to see the plastic surgeon I noticed a young woman and a man I had seen the day of my surgery. Vicki and I spoke with the couple while we all waited to see the same doctor. They were married and had three small children. She had the same surgery and also had the hereditary gene. Her family had a strong history of ovarian cancer. I know her experience will be quite different than mine, as she is so young. She was beautiful and very sweet. Her swept-up hair made her look like she was going to a high school prom. After a while I was called in for my appointment and we wished them the best.

The removal of the drains felt like long snakes being pulled out of me quickly. It was not painful, just peculiar. Afterwards, I began to have my expansions done. This required a shot of liquid saline to be added at each visit. Forty-eight hours after having my drains removed, I was able to shower. I felt like a human being again; what a relief.

Recovery presented challenges, but everything seemed manageable. Even the physical discomfort was easier to tolerate than I had anticipated. I expected to get back to most of my normal tasks soon.

The memorial service for my Uncle Leon was held sixteen days after my surgery. It was a special service that was sincere and personal—he would have approved heartily. Attending the service was important to me. Of course, everyone would have understood my absence. After the luncheon we were able to spend a brief time with the entire family.

Weeks ago, I would never have counted on being able to attend and this felt like a big accomplishment.

After surgery I could not drive for about four weeks, and I was particularly interested in doing that again. Before long things were back to what was usual. We survived.

Strange and Surprising

In the weeks following my mastectomy, I went for my post-op visits with both surgeons. I went for my first expansion with the plastic surgeon on September 3. It was slightly uncomfortable, but unnoticeable by the next day.

As the weeks passed, my friends were especially terrific about spending time with me and I received all kinds of thoughtful gestures. Ginny kept me walking and listened to the daily details about my experience. Vicki and I were in constant touch. Laura in her gracious style came by loaded with goodies. She gave me a blank journal and suggested that I might want to chronicle what I was going through. I had never kept a diary successfully before and I wasn't quite sure about that idea. She also brought a complete homemade dinner for us to enjoy. My friends were amazing!

Now, I was concentrating on recovery and really getting back to my new reality, or something like it. I became obsessed with boobs, and as I walked the streets of the city to my appointments I noticed each breast I passed along the way. Not in a sexual way, but in a critical way. I mentioned this to John. He simply said, "I hate breasts now." I understood. This has been difficult for my husband on many levels. It was understandable—all of this was a huge and unwelcome change.

The intimacy aspect of our relationship was one that I definitely had taken for granted and it had been seriously altered. Part of that is due to the time needed to recover from surgery. We will adjust; but this was more of an emotional strain than I ever imagined. *Good health and self-image are powerful things.*

I felt like I was wearing a hard corset that was too tight on me all the time. Lying on my side was close to impossible for a long time after surgery. Except for the pain of healing muscles and in some surrounding tissue, my chest has lost all feeling. My upper arms and underarms were mostly sore and achy, especially during the overnight hours.

Sleeping was uncomfortably for the first several months. I had never been a back sleeper, and it was actually painful on my lower back and buttocks to do so. Most nights I had to stay in our den propped up. I was getting up and constantly changing my position. Also I was going to the bathroom multiple times each night. This was a result of drinking large quantities of fluids to counter-act the pain medication's side effects.

I worried about John not getting enough sleep because of all this. The more I thought about that, the more I could not sleep. I had been given sleep-aide medication, but I was reluctant to use it regularly. My couch sleeping bothered John and became a touchy matter at times. Day times were much easier. We were trying hard but there were problems. Even so I think we managed fairly well.

John pitched in where he could. He helped me lift things of any real weight, and accompanied me to the food store. I truly appreciated what he was doing. He listened, but rarely asked me how I felt. I tried not to drive him crazy by complaining and obsessing, which I did not want to do anyway.

—⁂—

Soon after I returned to driving, Cara and I went to breakfast as a mini-celebration regarding that activity. At the end of our meal she announced that she wanted to talk to me about something important. "Just listen." she said, "Don't say a word until I am finished, OK?" I was braced for . . . I don't know what! Then, she continued to explain, "Anne and I have decided that we want to do something to remember how strong you were in handling this crisis. We think the three of us should get the same breast cancer tattoo. It would be a sign of solidarity." I was shocked by this idea, which caught me totally off guard.

At first I just laughed a little at this whole ploy. Anne has often taunted me about the possibility of getting a tattoo. Cara has never talked to me about an interest in this before, so this was more surprising and I told her, "You know I'm not a fan of having permanent things like that done to your body. I am afraid you might regret this someday." I felt like I had to exercise some parental responsibility here and not encourage this mistake.

She reminded me about how little she asks me for in general, and how responsible she is most of the time, and that she is a "good kid." I was in complete agreement on all those points. Then she said, "Mom, it will always remind me of your courage and how strong you have been. That means a lot to me. You know, this may be *my* issue someday."

I was blown away. She stated her case, and did an excellent job of it. I took a deep breath, and told her, "I'm not ready to go along with this idea, but it will be kept under consideration for now." I did appreciate what she said and her effort. Cara is a determined person, yet very respectful and cautious. She knew a tantrum or fuss would never work. I was pretty impressed and it was difficult to not give in.

By the way, this is not the same issue regarding Anne and the BRCA gene because she was adopted, so she can't inherit this from me. Since this is the first mention of this, let me just say Keith is also adopted. We consider Cara our (biological) bonus child.

Anyway, I told John later on about the entire conversation between Cara and me. As he listened his eyes widened with an expression that conveyed he did not think it was a good idea. Cara has reminded me once or twice more on the subject. It is a careful little nudge.

MORE DECISIONS

My pal Ginny was fantastic about stopping by often. We went for frequent walks in my neighborhood, and she always let me determine how far we would go. Her company helped push me to keep exercising. Sometimes we had tea and we just chatted. I sent her a note to express how much her interest and help has meant to me. We had grown much closer. Timing in life can be awfully funny sometimes.

As my body healed it became clearer that some things had changed drastically. Sleeping improved a bit as the plastic surgeon told me it would. He was sure that my discomfort was not caused by the expanders; he felt it was from the actual healing from surgery. I wasn't completely convinced.

However, I developed a phobia regarding the expanders. I kept worrying about a leak. This idea concerned me because I have learned that once you have implants any such problem requires a surgery to replace them. Such a problem would be unlikely; but I realized that the conditions of the implants are a new and lasting concern for me.

The expansions went well on September 15 and 22. Each time the nurse found the metal port in the expander by using a magnet. Then she injected a shot full of saline fluid enlarging the tissue expander itself. It was quick and painless. The first night I felt a tightness develop and a day or two later that was gone. The expanders looked as though I stuffed two little bowls under my skin, which was not a particularly natural shape. Yes, I did realize no one else noticed this.

The plastic surgeon decided on the size implants. I was glad that I was going to be smaller as they felt very unnatural. Larger implants did not seem like a better solution especially for sleeping. I expected that the doctor knew best. There were going to be four expansions and then some time before the job was completed. This doctor never asked about how I felt nor had any personal discussion. He was aloof and silently intimidating; and so I hadn't summoned up the nerve to ask or tell him much, either. Maybe he doesn't even know how uncomfortable these expanders are; I bet other patients have a similar rapport with him.

It felt like forever before I got my results back on the evaluation of my tumor regarding chemotherapy. I had an appointment to see the breast cancer oncologist to discuss that and my future course of action. I was sure chemo was *not* needed in my case. I was very uncomfortable that I needed to see this particular doctor at all. Obviously, I was on another planet!

September 23, 2009 I met with the oncologist for the first time. Her young "fellow-doctor" came in first; he was with a young woman he was teaching. They examined me and spoke with us for a while. Afterward they left the room and returned in a few minutes with the oncologist.

I was expecting to meet Dr. Death. Instead this tiny, dynamic woman entered the examination room. Her petite frame and stylish shoes, along with her thick, long hair gave the impression she was younger than she later confessed she was. She had a warm smile and a sincere, casual demeanor, which made me feel oddly at ease.

The oncologist introduced herself as she shook John's hand first. Then she congratulated Vicki on being a "survivor." She walked toward me and did the same. The doctor spoke to my sister and asked her questions about her experience. She knew Vicki's original doctor well and shared similar sentiments of her loss, which pleased my sister very much.

The oncologist told me, "You are doing the things that I would have wanted you to do considering the facts." She commended me on showing my daughters my courage, and said, "It is a great lesson for them." Her comments made me feel good. As she examined me we were given more information.

Next, we all met in her office. The fellow and his student talked with us for a while. After a few minutes the oncologist came and joined the party. She explained some of what they had gone over with us again. Then she explained how chemo works. She showed me the results of my test. It came back with results right on the border, considered a "grey area." The oncologist said, "It is not perfectly clear how beneficial this treatment is in this case."

The test also showed that the tumor was larger than we thought. It was actually 1.4 cm, which gave the doctor pause as she read the new information aloud. This did not affect her recommendation.

"You have done so much already and you are committed to removing the ovaries next." she said adding, "There are no guarantees with any of this. If, after *everything* you have done—even one cell has escaped and started to develop somewhere in your body, this therapy might possibly save you."

You don't know what works, when you do more than one thing. You only know when despite everything, nothing works. There are a small percentage of patients who fall in that category.

This was all too much. I was definitely in shock! The chemo treatments would make at least a six-month extension in my journey. I would receive an IV treatment of the standard CMF chemotherapy (Cytoxan, Methotrexate and 5-FU) every three weeks. There would be eight treatments over the six months. Of course, there might be delays during that time.

If I was sick, or my blood work was not right before a treatment, the schedule was subject to change. I remembered the plastic surgeon told me, "Surgery won't take place for at least two months past the completion of chemotherapy." He added that there might be a conflict with his and the gynecologist's schedule, causing more delay. The chemo did not sound like an attractive option and I was unhappy about it. I found the whole idea almost unbearable. We had to think this one over.

The doctor appeared very understanding, but insisted on us making appointments for two weeks later. One was another meeting with her for a quick exam and a second consultation. The second appointment later that same day was for my first chemo treatment. The doctor explained I could cancel that one even as late as that morning.

I liked this doctor; but I was quite confused about what to do. She made sure to point out to me that the treatments were better than when Vicki had hers years before. They had learned in time that less chemo was needed to do the job. The doctor was adamant the chemotherapy would be better than I was imagining. She told me to call with any questions.

Noticing our reservations the doctor said, "Amy, it is your decision. Whatever you decide, I won't lose any sleep over your decision." Chemo was her recommendation and if we were opposed to following it, she would respect that. I mostly understood how she meant it, but her choice of words at this time was confusing me.

As we discussed my medical history at length during this consultation, the doctor said she thought a thorough blood workup was needed. They scheduled me to do that right after we finished with the oncologist. Vicki needed to leave early in order to attend an event that afternoon. We told her we did not need her to stay longer today. My sister finally agreed and left us. Our plan was to finish up then, take a cab to John's office, and get a ride home with one of John's co-workers. We left after the blood work was completed.

It was September 23 and still quite warm. Both John and I were starving and our first order-of-business was lunch. After that we started to walk as we felt it would be good for us. Before long we walked so far it seemed silly to get a cab. It was lovely to be out and about. Eventually we walked through Central Park. We kept going almost pretending this was the best day; and that it was not simply that we were numb.

It finally hit us that we were crazy-hot and the last few blocks were a bit uncomfortable. Jeepers, I had surgery six weeks earlier; and now I was walking across Manhattan. Was John trying to kill me? It seemed incredible that I was able to do this long walk considering what I had been through recently. *It was a good lesson about how even a small amount of time makes such a big difference.*

We stopped at John's office and he checked up on things there. His co-workers were kind in extending their concerns and best wishes. Then John and I stepped back out and crossed the street. We bought ice-cream bars and sat as we looked over the Hudson River. Actually, we were barely conscious of where we were. After a while we returned to the office for our ride home.

I remember thinking that it had been both a good-day and a bad-day. There was another big decision to be made. Again, no one else could tell me what I should do. This became the most difficult decision for me. I kept flip-flopping back and forth. The risks seemed both small and huge at the same time. What if I put myself, my body, my husband and family through *all this* and did not follow through with the chemo? Perhaps everything I have done, and still plan to do is *not* enough? If, that same breast cancer returns—will I then feel that I might have been one of the lucky persons that chemo takes care of by killing any dividing cancer cells? Remember, there are patients that none of the previously mentioned steps will help in the end.

This whole deal was pretty much of a gamble. I usually cannot afford to gamble and it is not my style. If the doctor had said that my score indicated a definite benefit and need, the answer would be easier and much more palatable. The idea of introducing my body to chemotherapy was in itself frightening. This choice was completely distressing.

I had my last expansion on September 29. In a rare extended conversation I told the plastic surgeon about my chemotherapy dilemma and he only said, "The delay is not a problem, there will be more healing during that time and that is fine." Finally, we were able to elicit a smile from him, which was a large accomplishment on our parts. He actually joked with us and both Vicki and I thought it worth noting. I had asked him as he was bolting out the door, "Do you need to know which implant

I am choosing?" His quick reply was, "No, and *I* won't lose any sleep over that." He thought himself quite clever and he turned to us with a big smile. OK, it wasn't that big, but it was a smile!

We patted ourselves on our backs for that out-of-character moment. This little slip of his was worth the trip in. I was asked to call his office and let them know what decision I made about the chemo. I was still "on the fence" . . . what to do, what to do?

My sister-in-law Rita had heard what was happening from her sister Mary. Rita called because she wanted me to speak to her friend who is an oncology nurse. Rita is John's younger sister, and I have known her friend since they both were young girls. Her friend has probably been an oncology nurse for over twenty-five years. I phoned her soon after speaking with my sister-in-law. I shared lots of information that I had been given and she agreed with everything. She cautiously said, "If I were in the same position I would most likely take the chemo." I asked her some questions and I was sure she was being honest. It was sweet of her to try and reassure me.

Finally, I told myself chemo was probably the best thing to do. I still anticipated it would be rougher than the doctor and her staff portrayed it to be. I equated chemo with poison—right or wrong, I was scared. I am by my nature a "glass-half-empty" kind of person. Now, I was fighting my normally negative side all the time. I wanted to make *this* decision with as much confidence as possible.

Two days before my first chemo appointment I had to call the oncologist who was unavailable and had to call me back. Meanwhile I had been trying to straighten out some things between my insurance company and the hospital for days. This is enough to drive anyone over the edge. By the time I spoke with my doctor I was having a meltdown.

I had concerns and I needed to discuss them with her before I went ahead. Never has anyone been more approachable, understanding and compassionate with me. She listened to my personal issues. Not for one moment did I feel that she was judging me in any way. This doctor did not minimize or dispute my feelings; she was kind and helpful. The bottom-line was that she did not want me to have any regrets. After reminding her about the comment regarding "not losing any sleep" over my decision she apologized for the phrasing, and made sure I understood her meaning.

The doctor said, "I understand how you could choose not to do the chemo. However, I operate on the side of caution." She felt it was a valid course of action in my case. She stated, "Your apprehension makes it impossible to start treatments this week. We will only go ahead with treatments if you are sure of your decision." She suggested that I take more time to think it over. She thought if I were to have chemo it had to be started within two weeks.

That night I thought it over and decided I had to go for it. I called my doctor's office early the next morning. I told them that I wanted to go ahead. I would understand if it were too late, but that I would like to come in as planned. It took a while for their return call. They told me I could keep my appointment and start the first treatment.

Again, John would not say what he thought I should do about the chemo. He just said he knew I would make the right decision. We have one medical philosophy in common, which is: For every intervention, there is always the chance *that* intervention will likely cause another issue. I really did get where his reservations were coming from. Everyone said they thought I made the right choice. At least I will never look back and think maybe I could have done more. That could be big. I needed a break already!

On October 7, Vicki and I went to my first treatment. The doctor examined me and we spoke a bit more. She let her nurse handle most of the details concerning the treatments, any possible side effects and diet. We talked about avoiding germs as much as possible. She suggested avoiding sick people and crowded places like malls. The nurse presented me with more papers to read. We had to wait until we were called into the chemo suite.

The facility was new and everyone seemed proud of the amenities. I was anxious to get everything over with, so I was not as impressed. Vicki on the other hand, remembered her own experience in comparison and she thought the new chemo suites were great.

One stroke of luck was that my nurse Ann was an absolute doll. Oddly enough, the nutritionist who spent time with us name was Cara: of all the possibilities, my daughters' names? I considered this a good sign. Ann went over most of the same things that the nurse had done earlier. Then she carefully explained the procedure before and during the entire process. She was very considerate and friendly, but she maintained a highly trained and efficient air. This put me at ease. Well, mostly.

I had to start by taking three anti-nausea pills and three steroid pills, which made the first work better. Then she started the IV. With each step Vicki asked which one was being administered? She just wanted to double-check that all was correct. Actually it was a triple check. Another nurse always comes in at the beginning to verify that all the medications are correct. So, I was triple-secure!

The whole treatment was completed in under an hour. They did give me more anti-nausea medicine to take home and a sleep-aide as well. I might not need these. They warned me that the medication might cause constipation. I took the pills home knowing that I would only take them if it was absolutely necessary.

The most important thing to remember was to drink lots and lots of fluids. They kept emphasizing the importance of that. I am not much on drinking large or even moderate amounts of liquids. This would take real effort on my part. Caffeine drinks did not count and generally needed to be replaced quickly by non-caffeinated ones. Water was preferable. Yuck.

I felt slightly odd, but definitely not sick as the day went on. I was exhausted in the evening and had a tough time even watching my Yankees that night. I think that it was more about my nerves than anything else. I drank like a fish! It likely was the most fluid I had ever had before. I awakened five times that night to go to the bathroom. Oh yeah, this was going to be challenging.

The next morning I was OK until after breakfast. The sleeping pill had been unnecessary, but now I was feeling a little queasy. After breakfast I had to take my first anti-nausea pill. I was committed to walking as many weekday mornings as we could. It seemed even more important now that treatments had started. Everything went fine. Walking was good and I did not feel any strain in exercising. Today my life was "normal." That was great.

It is difficult to describe; maybe I was concentrating too much on how I was feeling. My mouth had a funny taste and was dryer than usual. I used the recommended toothpaste and mouthwash to help with that.

The steroids obviously kicked in a day later. I had forgotten the nurses told me the steroids might have some effect on my energy level in a day or two. After my breakfast I started to put away the dishes from my dishwasher. I became sorely aware of how overcrowded and unorganized my kitchen was and I began to rearrange each shelf. Truthfully, I must have been half way through straightening all the cabinets before I gave my efforts any thought. It occurred to me that the steroids were likely responsible for this accomplishment. Straightening these cabinets had been a long neglected job, and I was pleased to have tackled it successfully. Boy, some extra energy would come in handy around here.

STARTING MY JOURNAL

My walking buddies were all away. Ginny went to Florida for a few days; and Vicki and my niece Jen were in Boston on business. Inexcusably, I had not gone for my walks.

As mentioned earlier, my friend Laura visited me one day shortly after my surgery in August. She brought a blank writing journal to record my experiences and thoughts. It seemed like a reasonable idea. Even then, I had already missed months of my experience. It is now further along as it is October of 2009. It was way back in May that I had my mammography. I have been thinking about writing, and this week felt like the perfect time to start.

It was easy for me to use the notebook from all my doctor's appointments. Those detailed notes allowed me to refer to facts and even comments from each meeting. I did not want to depend on remembering important information so I was very precise. After I received my friend's journal I also made separate notes. Those would be reminders of various items I wanted to include if, I decided to write. At first it was fun to figure out how to organize and get started. Obviously, I had lots to fill in before reaching present day. As this was the longest, single event and time period I ever focused on me, I had no difficulty in recalling my experience thus far.

With my buddies all away, I had a chunk of alone-time to spend on this effort. After writing constantly for several days, I completed writing about the first five months of my breast cancer journey. Finally I had it all down in black and white. I was comfortable this was a complete and accurate story. From now on, I will continue to makes entries as I see fit. This is exciting! It is both reflective and therapeutic to evaluate your feelings and actions. I can see all the support I have had over these months. Now, it's all there to remind me.

This project was so enjoyable that I began to think that maybe my children would benefit from being able to read it someday. I am not so regimented that I want to write every day, so I will continue as time and interest allow.

Since I am stuck home waiting to have a new furnace installed, writing is an ideal diversion to distract me from being annoyed. Normally this large expense would have upset me. Instead, I am mostly thankful that it did not happen in the dead of winter. OK, maybe I'm a little out of joint about it, but not like the old Amy would be. Amazing what a little perspective can do for you. I felt a little lucky that this problem was discovered now and I told John just that. He said, "Isn't it funny what we consider lucky these days?" Maybe, I just didn't care today; we needed heat and now we have it. *Cancer makes lots of things look different.*

In fact, I have been thinking how my crisis has altered many of my relationships and experiences. Vicki and I are enjoying a strengthened bond and her supportive encouragements are great reinforcements. The fact that she has been totally dependable and available has been fantastic. I haven't forgotten what a busy business woman she is. It is customary for my sister to stroll through the waiting room area while conversing with her associates and clients. Never does she display frustration or concern that this situation has created any stress or difficulty for her, which allows me to feel more comfortable.

This experience has also highlighted some funny things about my sister's habits for my observation and amusement. She has an acquired obsession with her daily tea: it is a particular order she requires every day from her favorite coffee shop. Vicki tends to order every food in her own unique way. This drink is really individualized even for her. It is a certain tea and a particular amount of water, which is placed in a larger cup than her actual order size. Then she has the sweetener amount altered, and two inches foamed skim milk added last. That probably is not even correct though I have heard the order so many times. My sister is definitely a "high maintenance" gal. Believe me, it makes a critical difference!

It is essential that we always have a lunch plan; a good thin-crust pizza with healthy toppings, or salad with dressing limitedly used on the side is the perfect complement to our chemo day. Vicki always manages to reinforce her philosophies on attitude, positive thinking and general dieting to me. She is a "piece of work" but I would not be able to manage without her help.

I often hear from people who are concerned about how I am doing and their interest lifts my spirits. I never thought that I had many friends. So, it is a pleasant surprise that this situation has brought me closer, and in more frequent contact with many people. It has shown me that even when you are not close to a person their kindnesses are very meaningful. I am ashamed to think of all the opportunities I have missed to do the same for someone else.

Mentioning all the specific ways this happened so far is impossible. Some examples are: neighbors who call or bring some homemade food to the door, a basket that arrives with flowers or goodies from a former job, visits from dear friends, cards and gifts from people—some of whom I really don't even know. Often the biggest efforts come from the least expected sources. Even my regular gynecologist phones randomly from time to time to inquire about how I am doing. It has been an overwhelming and amazing experience.

It is also apparent that my breast cancer crisis has impacted many people that I love and care for. Not just my immediate family circle. John's Aunt Betty is now almost ninety-three years old. Betty has been able to depend on me in lots of ways. Her daughters live a distance away and this has worked for all of them for a while. Things will have to change a bit as my recovery and making more time for my brother are my biggest priorities. Visits with Betty will be mostly over the phone for while. I know she will understand.

It is exactly two months since my mastectomy. I feel that things have gone better in many ways than I anticipated. I did things that might have seemed impossible had I thought about them after my surgery.

Best of all, our lives have continued along as usual. Keith and Cara began their school year in September without a hitch. Anne tells her friends, "We don't live in a cancer house at all." She means that things haven't really changed much. Once chemo was planned, I did some uncustomary early shopping. Cara and I bought her Halloween costume and accessories. Then we purchased some clothes to get her through the Sweet Sixteen parties coming up. I was not sure how the treatments would go, and I felt a little extra preparation would be wise.

There are some differences in the things that I often think of doing. Besides staying out of stores more than usual, movie theaters strike me as places to pick up nasty germs as well. I love to go see a current flick, but there won't many of those for a while. Cara's school is a place I particularly want to avoid. I skipped the routine "Back to School Night" for the first time. The idea of going room to room and seat to seat gave me the willies! These modifications are all fine and not terribly difficult. Perhaps it is easier for me to slow down a little, as I lead a fairly quiet life anyway. I'm determined go to the holiday concert and the school play no matter what!

I feel that my recovery has been good and for that I am extremely fortunate. My daily post-surgery exercises have paid off. I have full range of motion with some soreness. I can even get in and out of my Rutgers hooded sweat shirt and not feel as though I need to call for help. Once again I am reaching for things on the higher shelves in my kitchen. I am lifting items that are not too heavy. Unfortunately, the vacuum is not too heavy for me to use.

John came home with a cold. Several men in his small office had been sick earlier in the week. I expected this would be the case as they often pass these illnesses around. This tiny office with no windows and one bathroom makes avoiding such situations almost impossible.

The oncologist had given me the regular flu shot before I started chemo. Now I wanted to avoid even a cold. John had no time to get vaccinated and he could not get one while already sick. Keith came home to get the shot a couple of weeks ago, but instead got an antibiotic for a cold he could not shake. Cara was having either a cold or allergy symptoms, and it was not good for her to get a shot either. Anne said she might get one although she is adamantly opposed to such vaccines. I knew that it was unlikely to happen. I am worried even though I know it is a waste of time.

As required, I went for a mid-treatment blood test to check on my white cell count. Chemo can create low counts, which can lead to not fighting off infections. I went to a local lab. It seemed silly to go into the city for this little test. After my doctor received the report her nurse called me to say my count was low. She asked if I thought I might be sick. I felt good but she insisted I repeat the test in a couple of days.

I am getting neurotic watching John's cold get worse and I may have a touch of something starting. I hope not because that can delay my next treatment. Feeling well I called Ginny to go for a walk after my test. Later I went for second walk with Vicki. She had been away and this was our first meeting in many days. We went to the county park halfway between us. It was lovely out and I felt fine.

Laura called and postponed bringing lunch for Ginny and me tomorrow. She might be coming down with something and did not want to make me uncomfortable. We decided to try again next week. Maybe I'm making everyone paranoid. My concerns are about interruptions in my treatment schedule more than about how sick I might become.

I am making my family a little germ crazy, too. My lecturing about washing hands, keeping them away from the face, and not going close to anyone who appears sick in any way is constant. A simple cough or a sneeze is enough to make me suspicious. I have asked my family to emphasize the problem of bringing sickness into our home to their friends.

Anne is going to a wedding in Texas this coming weekend. Usually my main concern would be about her flying. Instead I keep thinking that people will go to a wedding sick or not. When I think of all the kissing and hugging it makes me crazy. Airports must be a great germ-fest also. Oh, what about the planes?

As I think of these things I'm taking advantage of the mild weather and I'm airing my house out. I am desperately trying to clean more to rid it of John's cold germs. Our house has not been disinfected like this for a long time. Hopefully I will avoid this cold and keep to my schedule.

Even with all the effort I woke up feeling a little something coming on. I was edgy and annoyed with myself. As much as I would try to deny it I was getting a cold.

My mood is not good as some decisions of the last couple of days are bothering me. First, my friend's mom passed away over the weekend and I am not going to the funeral. He said he understood. It is hard not to get physically close to those people who you want to console and speak with. Again, funerals attract people whether they are healthy or not. I didn't attend.

Today I'm feeling rather selfish and like a terrible person. Also I cancelled lunch with Laura again. Maybe I should have given it more time to be sure I wouldn't be better tomorrow? I am lucky if I have any friends left when this is all behind me!

The cutest little Boy Scout came to my door to do some fundraising this afternoon. Upon a look-see, I was surprised at the expensive items. Heck, I'm talking about gourmet popcorn. I looked to the bottom of the brochure to find a few nine-dollar items. I remarked, "Since I lost my job some months ago I'm very careful about how I spend my money." This little guy looked up and said, "Someone just bought three of these." He pointed to the forty dollar tub of popcorn. Obviously, my unemployment did not impress him at all. I told him to try me another time. Luckily he did not push me any further; I might have had to play the cancer-card next. I doubt that would have had any impact on him either. He was a man "on a mission."

After he left my front steps I thought, *Maybe I am a "bad" person.* Jeepers, I better get out and walk off some of my anxieties.

JUST KEEP GOING

About a week has passed since I wrote in this journal. I came down with a cold and I had two blood tests. The first one showed that my white cells were quite low. The doctor wanted the second one done as a precaution and that one was better. The nurse thought based on those results, I should be able to have my second treatment next week.

This year I invited Ginny to join Laura and me for my birthday lunch. Ginny's birthday is one week before mine, yet it always surprises her when I remember her day. I made lunch for us and as always we had fun and chatted up a storm together.

Laura had gifted me with a small bag of goodies. It is our version of *Oprah's Favorite Things*. I loved all these handpicked items: a pen, magnetic measuring spoons, breast cancer pink walking gloves, a powerful-tiny flashlight and a lovely silver angel pin. The angel has a pink breast cancer ribbon around her waist. When we get together there is a part of me that feels sixteen again. It was a great day with these friends.

Days later my actual birthday day, October 24, was quiet. John and I were not over our colds, and we cancelled plans to join Vicki and her husband Paul and my Mom and Irwin for dinner. John was not interested in coughing through everyone's meal and I agreed that he was right.

Cara had a busy Saturday which included helping out at the middle school play rehearsal. Later she accompanied her best friend who was getting ready for her big Sweet Sixteen bash. Even so, Anne and she found the time to give me a birthday present along with a scrumptious pumpkin ice-cream pie. Wow, I loved that! They bought me a beautiful silver engraved frame for the picture I had taken with me to the hospital of them with Keith. It was perfect.

Anne wrote the most touching card ever. She spoke of how proud they are of me. She mentioned how well they thought I managed to keep things "normal and positive." I will always treasure that card. Keith remembered to call me from school and that simple effort delighted me.

John had wanted me to shop for something with him. But, I thought it unnecessary and unwise to be among all the Saturday shoppers' germs. This fifty-seventh year should be . . . interesting at very least. I am feeling like my family made sure it was off to a good start.

Wednesday, October 28 I woke up more congested then I have been since I started with this cold. I was uneasy as this was chemo number two today. I had thought I was getting better yesterday and now I was not sure. I was more uncomfortable knowing how much Vicki hates being near sick people. It is a residual feeling from her chemo days. She is adamant about staying away from germs. She thought the doctor might not allow me to have this treatment and yet she had taken me in. I felt well enough to give it a try.

Due to heavy rains our trip was longer than ever before. The more I worried about coughing and sniffling—the more I felt the need to do so. The air in the car seemed to make me feel worse. Finally, the coughing fit I was fearful of came; Vicki remained calm. Thank God, we were able to stop for her tea on the way in to New York this morning! She was a trouper; Vicki simply decided no matter what else happened there was going to be a thin-crust pizza included in our day. She also decided on a different pizza for the next appointment day. This aspect of her personality surely lends itself to her general life's success.

We went in with fingers crossed. There I took another finger prick blood test. The doctor came and examined me and we spoke. She said she might have preferred me to wait; but my blood was reasonable and I had no fever and so I could continue. I was happy to keep going. Many of the people in the waiting room, the receptionist and even my doctor, had colds today. The doctor put me at ease with her usual warm manner. She did prescribe an antibiotic for me to take home. We were off to the chemo suite after a short wait.

I was happy to have the same sweet and efficient chemo nurse. Ann is from the city and is also a Yankee fan. Tonight is the first game of the World Series, so we were all excited. Even my sister is catching Yankee fever. Our conversation made the time go even faster. The treatment was a breeze and we were off for our pizza. We learned that if we go right away for my blood work from now on, we will save a lot of waiting time. Another thing to remember is that a cold is not critical, but *no fevers* are allowed at the office and chemo suites.

Additionally I cleared up some dietary concerns: No fresh mozzarella cheese is allowed when you are on chemo, however, cooked on pizza is fine. Dried fruits and nuts were OK, too. My internet information was different and this was a relief. Those non-exclusions will make life a little tastier!

As the "big things" become more overwhelming, the "little things" become more important.

The night of my chemo was not bad. I had a headache as I did the first time. As pleasant as they try to make the experience, it is still stressful in the end. The headaches may be as much from the stress as anything else. Again I felt more tired on the night of chemo. Drinking tons of fluids has remained difficult for me. No matter, the Yanks are playing Game 1 and maybe that will make things a little easier tonight. All is good.

Last night's game was a disaster! We lost. Oh well, we have got to keep going. My night was not awful, but I woke up several times. I was queasy and needed to take some anti-nausea medication. The next morning my extra energy from the pre-chemo medication kicked in. I had taken Cara to school at 7:15 in the morning, and went straight to the food store. When I returned home I called Ginny to join me for a walk. It may have been too much as I felt poorly after all that. My cold came back, but I should not complain. The day ended on a high note as the Yankees won Game 2. Yay, I'm feeling better already!

This weekend I felt crummy and still pounded from my cold. Not being able to shake this thing and worrying constantly about germs was making me irritable. I am starting to think that chemo may have been a mistake. I am annoyed by my cough which makes my ribs hurt and chest muscles sore. The expanders add to the discomfort. My ribs had bothered me before and after my surgery at times. Right before this cold they had finally gotten better. Now they were very painful again. A deep breath, or too much time on my side and I am really uncomfortable.

Having a bad case of cabin-fever I desperately needed to break out. A few days later I felt a little better and I ran out to shop for a present. Vicki and Paul's fortieth anniversary is this weekend. We have pretty much stopped exchanging such gifts. However, this is a nice milestone and I wanted to find something for them this year to show some special appreciation.

I felt up to running to the quietest mall nearby. Vicki and Paul don't need any of the traditional keepsake gifts. I decided that after forty years it is all about comfort, and I found each of them a great sweater. It was satisfying to be on this little jaunt. I ran home and immediately wrapped the presents.

Later, Vicki called and asked me to join her for a walk in the park that we most often exercise at. Her sister-in law had something for me and wanted to meet us there. It seemed odd to me. Vicki thought it might have something to do with a church group. We all met and had a nice walk.

It turned out that the gift was quite unique and special. It was from a Catholic church's Prayer Shawl Ministry, a group of women who pray for someone while they are making a shawl for them. The shawl is a symbol of God's love, comfort and protection. The idea alone touched me. None of these people even know me. The note attached aptly expressed the purpose of this gift. Though not formally religious in any way, I do feel that I am somewhat spiritual. I knew it was a blessing to receive this gift. It reminds me of how much love and support I have received. It is a soft neutral green color, which I particularly like. Wow, what a kindness!

Just for the record the Yanks won Games 3 and 4 this weekend in Philadelphia. That was exciting! They can wrap it up there or come home and do it here in New York, the first year in their new stadium. Earlier this season this all seemed impossible. The Yanks battled through the rough beginning of the season and came back strong. They have the most likeable team they have had in years and it has been fun watching them. You have got to have "faith."

The weekend was busy between baseball games, my sister's anniversary and Halloween. Wow, we felt like "normal" people. John and I thought we could join Vicki and Paul at a restaurant over the weekend with Mom and Irwin. Saturday I woke fully intending to go out, but by the afternoon I had stomach cramps that forced me to stay home. It may have been the chemo, or maybe the antibiotic was also bothering me. I began feeling sorry and upset for myself that I was not able to be tougher.

Later that night, I settled down to watch Game 5. It was clear from the beginning that it was not the Yankees' night. The good news was that Game 6 would bring them home. It won't be an easy or sure win. Go Yanks! They had one day off. They needed a break and so did I.

Halloween was unusually quiet for a Sunday holiday. Every time children came to our door it reminded me of how fast time goes by. It felt just like yesterday when we walked our young children carefully around gathering up all the goodies. Heck, it also seems like not long ago I, myself, was trick-or-treating for hours and with no parent chaperone. When my bag was filled, I ran home to get another one for collecting more treats.

We did not worry about "bad candy" back then so, Halloween was a big score! I can still see my dad's face as he looked over the bounty and he made his personal selections. Come to think of it, John does the same thing.

Good, with this holiday over the rest of this year should fly by. All of this will become a blip on my screen. Yes!

CRISIS AND CELEBRATION

I ran out to get more bloodwork taken this morning. The results were important to me as this cold was still hanging on and now, I have a fierce pain in my chest from coughing. I am pretty sure that I pulled a muscle. I ran around doing my usual local errands. I figure that if I can do all this, I shouldn't complain about how things are going.

When the mail came I heard from Carol, our high school friend. Her notes are always just what I need. She also sent a book written by a breast cancer survivor. Other mail included a card from my former next-door neighbor. These gals brought a smile to me and I felt better. I was planning to settle-in and looked forward to Game 6 of the World Series. Go Yanks!

November 4, ended up totally different than I could ever have expected. Let me tell it this way, so as to separate the best from the worst. I received some terrible news, which I will expand on in a moment. I will say that I did watch the game that evening with a heavy heart. The Yankees won the World Series! This was put into a different perspective due to other events. I was still happy for this team, which I had watched faithfully all season. When they reached their goal it was fulfilling. I was delighted to see their pride and joy as they celebrated together and with their fans. It was great!

I have to take a few steps back here; I had tried to reach my sister at various points today. She was either not reachable, or when I did make contact Vicki said she could not talk. She was strange and I was worried that I had just taken too much of her time lately. Was all hell breaking loose . . . I didn't really know what was going on. I was not upset, but I was concerned because something felt wrong.

Meanwhile, I got a call from my doctor's nurse, who was not happy to hear about my lingering cold and was concerned about the pain in my chest. She spoke with the doctor and they told me to come to the hospital to get a chest x-ray in the emergency room. They wanted to be sure that it was not pneumonia or anything more serious.

Honestly, I was certain I had pulled a muscle coughing. John was just on his way home from his work day, and I did not want him to turn around to go back to the city tonight. Admittedly, I wanted to see the game and this idea did not sit well at all.

I called Vicki to see if she would be able to take me into the city tomorrow morning. She could not and apologized. I told her it was not a problem. John said he saw no reason to run in tonight, either. He would drop me off there on his way to work tomorrow and I could call him when I was through. My doctor's nurse was somewhat annoyed and said, "Do your best to get in as soon as possible." Instinctively I knew this would be fine.

Vicki called back a short time later. What she blurted out in tears was unbelievable. A friend of hers had been in a horrendous accident. This is a brilliant, dynamic, extremely attractive and kind human being who literally "had it all." He was taken to the hospital in critical condition. It was a frightening and awful situation; and a difficult few days for many people who cared deeply about him. Things are grave at best. We are all praying for a miracle.

My sister was totally distraught about her friend and I shared her anguish. It was difficult for Vicki to share the situation with me. She finds it almost impossible to speak about anything negative that might happen. Sometimes, you just cannot believe what is happening. It is an awful feeling when there is absolutely nothing that you can do to help someone. My sister needs to be close by supporting her friend along with his family right now.

The next morning I directed my focus back to me. John and I went to the emergency room and after a while, he left for work. As expected I was there for eight hours. I had lots to think about from the night before. I waited for my x-ray, doctors and eventually a CAT scan. As I watched the activity and people around me, I kept thinking how weird life can be. As I looked around the hospital I watched all the people who were battling their own health crisis. It is too heartbreaking and frustrating that any of these things happen. I am quite aware that I am very fortunate.

Yesterday all I could think about was how much I wanted the Yankees to win the World Series. Now, this was put into perspective by something so completely unexpected and shocking.

My day was long, and I finally was discharged knowing my lungs were clear and I had no clots. The doctor thought I most likely had pulled a muscle and sent me home with a new antibiotic. She reminded me that my resistance was lower because of the treatments. Then she told me to get rest, drink fluids and stay out of crowds.

I felt certain more exercise would be beneficial. The winter months were going to be challenging. I called John and we went back home.

After about a week, the person we have been so concerned about thankfully has pulled through. There will be needed time to recover, but this was great news! All the commotion concerning him has been exhausting. My inner voice is definitely telling me to redirect my focus on *my* own better health again.

HEADING INTO
THE HOLIDAYS

This week marks three months since my mastectomy. It's mid-November and the weather is starting to make walking outside less appealing. My two walking companions are better than I am about continuing outdoor exercise. I either will walk inside at a mall early in the morning, or I will reintroduce myself to my treadmill. I will miss their companionship, the fresh air and sunshine. Ginny is definitely not into being inside. Vicki is willing to try mall walking. However, she is determined not to spend too much time in the stores after opening time. Her germ phobia is on guard as we head into the holiday season. We will try and meet before the stores are opened.

I want to remain committed to the physical exercise which will help control my weight through treatments. My oncologist said, "Patients often gain about ten pounds or so, mostly because they feel entitled to some extra treats. Also, if you feel more tired you may not be as active during this time." I am being pretty conscientious at controlling this reasonably well.

I have given up sugar in coffee and tea. While on chemo I cannot use honey and I definitely miss that in my tea. I have cut back on my white foods consumption. I am far from rigid regarding my diet, but getting better. At this point my weight has been maintained, and the trick will be getting through the holiday overindulgence.

Today's mail brought another letter from my childhood friend Colette. Our moms lived across the street from each other for about fifty-five years. Her mom moved to a nursing home recently. Colette and I know one another since about age one-and-a-half years old. We parted ways when Anne was a toddler. We hadn't talked until her dad passed away about five years ago and I attended his wake. Her parents were great to me when I was growing up. Living across the street from each other, I was always in their house. They even included me on many trips to the shore during summer vacations. Colette's mom was a professional seamstress and when the time came she made my wedding gown. So, there is history here.

Colette heard of my diagnosis from my mom writing to her mom. She has been sending random notes to me ever since. Experiencing a serious health crisis of her own a few years back, Colette is very compassionate about such events. We continue to correspond and I am enjoying this relationship. Life is funny, isn't it?

I definitely think that connecting with people is important. Being un-techno-savvy, e-mails do not suit me. Hand written notes and letters are best for me. I love that. Too bad my handwriting hasn't improved with age or circumstances. I keep a basket in our living room filled with cards and miscellaneous gifts received since my surgery. I find it heartwarming to know they are there to remind me of all the support I have received. Once in a while, I will pick up some and reread the sentiments.

We expect Keith to come home for the weekend. Rugby obligations have kept him very busy. He has a rotator cuff injury he received in the last game. I have been concerned with his playing this particular sport as the game is rough and there is little or no equipment worn. This is one time I hated being right. He is passionate about rugby and is determined to return to it soon. I miss him and John definitely misses the male companionship when Keith is not around.

When our son arrives he will find a little comfort food waiting for him. I have made a big pot of my homemade chicken soup, "Jewish penicillin," and it smells delicious! It also sounds like a good remedy for my cold, which is still with me as well.

Cara just called with some news. She got the understudy role for one of the leads in this year's high school production. She had an understudy role last year—both are real compliments to her talent considering that she is only a sophomore. It means a lot of work with little glory. The part is already double-cast, so it is unlikely that she will step in during an official performance. It is still great experience for her. She is also double-cast in a small lead role for some of the performances. She seems pleased. I am amazed she can do any of this. She is better than she realizes and watching her perform is always fun for us. Today is a very good day!

November 18 was my third chemo day. Vicki and I finally got with the program. First we stopped to get bloodwork done at the blood lab there. Then we headed up to the doctor's appointment. I was feeling pretty good. The doctor entered the room with surprising information. My white cell count had plummeted down. She could not allow the treatment to be done today. I was extremely disappointed. She was ordering special booster injections for me. They would bring the white cell count up. I got one injection at the office and was told to have another one the next day. We rescheduled the chemo for next week.

It seemed silly to go back into the city tomorrow for the quick injection. The doctor told me to either give myself the shot or get someone else to help me. I cannot even watch injections break the skin. I get the willies, big-time! Luckily, I knew two neighbors with nursing backgrounds, and I was certain one of them would be able to help.

My niece Jen wanted us to come by her apartment. That sounded like a great way to make the trip in to New York worthwhile today. She has lived in the city for some time, but this was my first opportunity to see her digs. We drove to the Lower East Side; a young, energetic area that seemed ideal for her. I really liked her studio apartment. Now, I can picture her at home in her own environment.

Jennifer suggested a restaurant nearby. I followed her lead and ordered one of the "specials." We chilled out a while enjoying what was left of the afternoon. I'm glad we spent time with Jen. She is a huge proponent of a healthy lifestyle and has helped educate my sister. They are trying to exercise their influence on me, but I have a longer way to go. That's an understatement!

The next day I experienced muscle pain from the shot yesterday. I was having anxiety over the at-home injections. Laura was coming by for a visit before her shift at the hospital where she works. We got so caught up with lunch and chatting that I forgot to take the shot out of the refrigerator early enough for it to reach room temperature. Laura had to get to work and we decided to skip the injection.

I could not believe I forgot about the shot. Immediately I made calls to my neighbors, who are both nurses. I expected one would be able to help me out and the first to call back was the lucky winner.

Loretta, who lives right across the street from us called me and was agreeable about this job. Since I don't know her very well I felt as though it was a bit of an imposition. She couldn't have been more gracious. The injection was easily administered and we talked for a while. She offered her assistance in the next months. This is a blessing. My neighbor is very nice, and I think this may actually give us an opportunity to get to know each other better.

By the way, this shot does not enter a vein and instead it goes into soft tissue, which does not hurt much. I hope this second booster shot will be sufficient to get me through chemo on Monday. Next week is

Thanksgiving. The doctor wanted me to get chemo a few days before the holiday. She thought it would pretty much guarantee a trouble-free day, which seemed like a good plan.

The injections had some side-effects of their own making me feel achy. I experienced a strong headache, general bone aches and the strangest, severe breast bone pain. Thank goodness they had warned me of this, or I might have made a visit to the emergency room about this strange and intense pain.

Cara was home today with a fever. This is going to be a tough winter. I am telling myself to remain calm.

Monday, November 23, my chemo appointment went without a hitch. My blood count had taken a huge jump and I was good to go. My only complaint is that my nurse was not Ann. This other nurse was efficient, but lacking in any personality. I think that a smile and some light pleasantry should be a basic part of the prescription. Perhaps, I need to have more compassion. Maybe she was not having her best day, either.

Vicki and I watched TV until the treatment ended about forty-five minutes later. Between bloodwork, seeing the doctor, waiting for the treatment, having the chemo, and waiting afterwards to set up the next appointment this takes two-three hours to complete an appointment. Next was our pizza lunch and then our chemo day was concluded. Later I realized the headache I got the first two times was missing. However, this time I also did not get the energy boost the next morning or two. But I felt fine and was looking forward to the holiday on Thursday.

My sisters-in-law, Mary, Rita and Barbara, were kind enough to take over the holiday this year. Thanksgiving had been relegated to our home in the last few years. Ah, the blessings keep coming. It is the one day we count on to get together with Rita and her three children and ours. She lives out in west Jersey and between all their schedules and ours; it is a rare and welcomed day.

Rita hosted this day for years, until her husband Jerry died of an aggressive cancer several years ago. He was a fun-loving, large teddy-bear of a guy. Jerry was the person that helped keep us all together, even through the rough spots that develop in all families. Jerry left us all too soon. I believe he would be pleased to know we are all sharing the holiday.

As all the children become older these occasions are more relaxing. The days of worrying about how they are all getting along, where they are and what they are up to are over. Instead we sit talking and listening to their stories and allow them to make fun of us. It is quite clear that all of them are convinced that we, the older folk, are "out-of-it." It is probably true and so, it's OK.

John's brother Tom and his wife were hosting this year in their new home nearby. Barbara had said she was looking forward to using her new space to entertain more comfortably. I was relieved for this consideration. Mary was happy, too. Not only was she not hosting this holiday; but it was a milestone birthday for her on that same day. Turning sixty and going crazy with holiday preparations was not a winning combination in anyone's mind. It just seemed wrong. This year we were all looking forward to being together at the other Dempsey's home.

The only problem on this holiday was my brother's situation. Garry is now so difficult to manage that we couldn't bring him to join us as usual. Instead Mom and Irwin visited him at his group home earlier in the day. Vicki, Paul and Jennifer went by to see him later and before they went to dinner at a restaurant. We planned to have a visit over the weekend.

My brother has lost the use of three limbs, and having swelling in all of them was an additional concern. Although he is small, it is nearly impossible to move him. Getting him in and out of one of our vehicles with his wheelchair is not possible either. Without a special vehicle with a lift or ramps there are serious obstacles. He has issues with using the bathroom, too. We have not figured all those logistics out. He is disappointed, but knowing that this is a different year for me, he also understands. His spirits remain fairly good most of the time. His corny puns are as plentiful as ever. He has an amazing memory and always has a joke or two for us.

Thanksgiving was a pleasant day with all the aunts and myself helping out. As always Anne was terrific in lending a hand and did her part. I think considering I have had three treatments I managed particularly well. We had a cake and some presents for Mary to celebrate her birthday modestly. Hosting would have been too much for me, but I did my best to help out. Even that little extra work caused me to feel exhausted the next day.

Sunday John, Keith, Cara and I went to visit Garry. Truthfully, I am embarrassed to admit that I don't go to his group home often. It always puts me in a funk. The other residents are very nice, but I believe Garry to be the highest functioning. When I see him there, I see him as a member of this unique group with limited abilities and vastly different temperaments. When I see him on his own, he is just my brother.

Garry was so delighted to have us over. He sat propped up in a chair with his horribly, swollen legs raised on a hassock in his bedroom. My brother was happy surrounded by his immense Coca-Cola collection, and the photos of friends and family displayed all around him. Garry is the most personable and kindest person you would ever want to meet. Without exaggeration he knows people everywhere he goes. All of his mementos make you well aware of how much he is loved. As usual one of his favorite TV shows was on; it was an *Andy Griffith Show* rerun—a classic.

My brother has been through so much. His life is simple. He shares his home, his work-life, and all his activities, asking for very little in return. He loves to be with people, tell jokes, eat, dance and listen to music. His job is a great source of pride; he enjoys his work and his co-workers. Garry is the receptionist at the workshop offices at the Arc, an organization for people with intellectual and developmental disabilities. He also has a girlfriend. What he gives to everyone and everything he does is amazing. He is a very special person and a role model in many ways.

Garry's crisis is so much more serious than my own. The quality of his life has drastically deteriorated. There are more medical appointments coming up. We are hoping to get some answers about his condition, and interested to find something that can be done for him. We are all very worried and scared.

A couple of days ago I suggested skipping the Christmas tree this year. My family all reacted strongly against that idea. I thought it was a huge project, and I felt less interested in decorating knowing we won't do much entertaining this year. I was overruled. With Keith home for Thanksgiving, our artificial tree was set up on Saturday, which John appreciated.

Earlier in our marriage John and I decorated the tree together. When the children came along it seemed easier to make the tree something for them to look at and not touch. John kept them busy while I took care of the job. It became my present to my family. They tease me endlessly now about not having been allowed to help decorate the tree. Actually, I think they love to give me "the business." This job is therapeutic for me. Maybe it's my artistic nature; however, I'm a fanatic about finding the right spot for all these treasures. The kids think I am obsessed and laugh at how careful I am. If they wanted to help now, it would be fine. Yes, I might move some ornaments around later, and I recognize this is one of my bigger quirks.

The "good news" is we have great ornaments for each child to inherit a tree full of these beautiful treasures someday. There are handmade ones, gift ornaments, mementos, expensive and inexpensive ones. The tree displays our interests in guitars, drums, the Yankees, baby ornaments and more. There are those special ornaments from different times and places we want to always remember. It may not sound different from most everyone else's, but it is always exceptional.

Our artificial tree goes up when it's most convenient and stays until it becomes embarrassing. The tree got me into "the holiday spirit." The decorating of the rest of the house took another few days.

In the end, we have a warm and inviting holiday home. I always include a Menorah and dreidels for the Jewish holidays. We light the candles every night during that holiday. We don't want to give off a religious-vibe, but we respect our interfaith family. Maybe, this is what happens when a non-practicing Jew hooks up with a non-practicing Catholic?

My family is Jewish, but we never attended services. However, my father's fairly religious family exposed me to celebrating some Jewish holidays as a child. John came from a strong Catholic upbringing, but he stopped practicing when he went away to college and never found his way back. My folks were never upset that John was not Jewish. However, when we started dating John's mom was more uncomfortable that I was non-practicing in my religion than about me being Jewish. It may have taken her a while to get used to me, but ultimately we were fond of each other. Sadly, my mother-in-law passed away early in our marriage.

John and I have tried to raise our children to respect people for the way they choose to live, be it spiritual or not. We appreciate the community and positive reinforcement that formal religious practice offers. Yet, we both take exception to exclusion and lack of tolerance that is sometimes the result of any group.

WHO'S BEEN
NAUGHTY OR NICE?

Our children have been warned that this Christmas is going to be a little different. There are more money concerns. It has been a trying year, with both my layoff from work and my medical issues; Keith not getting much work during last summer; the economy's effect on John's company and so on. In addition, our children understand I am not going to spend the usual amount of time searching for gifts that this holiday often requires.

Anne really never asks for anything in particular. Keith always knows what he wants and gives me a list with quite a range of options. Cara is reluctant to make requests because she is practical and realistic and she knows I am even more so. John is either very specific about what he wants or he wants nothing. They are really not so difficult and are always reasonably happy in the end.

Although we are not major gift-givers, we all do our best to make the day special for each other. With the tree up and all the decorations in place, I was giving thought to how the shopping would go. Since I was committed to spending much less time in germ-ridden malls, efficiency was my game. I was starting to plan my strategy.

My friend Marian came by today for a couple of hours. She brought me a vase that her daughter made filled with flowers. I loved the vase. Her daughter suffers from MS and that mosaic vase will always remind me of her courage and strength. Marian also brought some dried fruits and nuts for me. I did not have the heart to tell her that I was having terrible issues with my mouth and tongue from the chemo. My tongue was swollen and sore, and my teeth felt like knives. Later I would call the doctor. I knew something had to be done to help these problems. Her goodies would be enjoyed another day.

The oncology nurse told me, "The mouth issue is a common side effect." She prescribed a special mouthwash that I could get at my pharmacy. She would call in the prescription right away. She also suggested that spicy foods are to be avoided. Food and drink brought to room temperature is also helpful and less aggravating. The nurse instructed me not to swallow any of the mouthwash. I was anxious to give this a try.

I spoke with my mom and she offered to pick up the medication for me on her way out to dinner. I was glad to have this help. I was out of sorts, cold in my own home and out of steam. Except for having my sister take me into the city, I haven't had to be dependent on others and I am thankful about that. Yet, it is nice to know that I have plenty of people who are there for me if needed. The thick, pink mouthwash did the trick. It was expensive and more important, immediately effective. What a relief!

My mom called later in the week and let me know Garry was receiving a special honor at the annual dinner-dance fundraiser for the non-profit organization he works for in two days. He has worked there for over twenty-seven years starting in the workshop, where many other intellectually and developmentally challenged adults are also employed. After some years, his great personality led them to promote him to the official greeter and receptionist. He has been an outstanding employee and they were presenting him with a special award.

Garry has been a strong and outspoken advocate for the rights of people with special needs and an extraordinary person. My dad was a volunteer for the Arc in the early days, and later became an administrator for this organization in another county in N.J. Dad would have been delighted to hear his son was being awarded on this occasion. Vicki and Anne joined Mom and Irwin to help celebrate this event.

I declined as I wanted to stay away from the crowd in this flu season. Mostly, I wanted to avoid the emotional aspect of this evening. I am an easy crier and even the thought of this night makes me fall apart. I could not handle it right now. I felt guilty about this; and I am pleased Anne insisted on representing us instead. Deep down, I knew I would regret this decision.

The evening was fantastic. Anne taped the presentation for us all to see. Garry's speech has been affected by his illness making it nearly impossible to understand his acceptance of the award. My brother has touched so many people deeply, and he is adored. It was lovely to see him shine even now. We do not know what is exactly happening regarding his health, but everyone is very disturbed by what we can see. Generally, he has been able to maintain his good spirits and gentle demeanor.

It is so important that they chose to honor him at this time. He was overwhelmed and quite pleased by this presentation. When his boss read its inscription it described him perfectly with love and admiration. We are so proud of him.

It has been days since I made an entry in my journal. Last week I imposed on my kind neighbor Loretta to give me five days of injections. Each day she came home from work and came straight over to help me out. We talk about lots of things in these brief times. We both have adopted children and biological children. Both she and I gave birth to our youngest child in our forties. Loretta has been a doll about helping me and I am indebted to her for this contribution to my care. She is a lovely, open and casual woman. She has been my neighbor for a few years and now we are finally becoming friends—another bonus.

Overall the injections are tolerable. I experience muscle and bone aches sporadically on two of the five days. Thank goodness, I did not have more of the severe breast bone pain this time. That was too weird. I am not conscious of the injections' effect on me. They certainly worked last time and hopefully, they will be effective again. Boosting the white cell production in your blood helps fight off illnesses and improves your resistance.

Feeling pretty good in general I decided to get out and try to accomplish some Christmas shopping. We told everyone outside our immediate family not to buy John and me anything this year. We were cutting out all those extra gifts. That was going to make my life so much simpler.

Keith simplified my search greatly. He had given me all the information required to order specific items on the Internet for him. He was in rugby heaven. I lucked out for Anne as in two stops I found some beautiful clothes for her. I bought what I thought she would like and needed, but would never treat herself to. Cara was also getting clothes, and I broke down and went to her favorite stores at a mall I rarely shop at another afternoon. Two stops and I found some great things for her. I was pleased with my purhases. Then I purchased a variety of gift cards so that all three could make some personal selections.

John was the most difficult to complete this year. I ended up buying him some CDs, a nice wool scarf for his dress coat, and a helmet for rollerblading, which he occasionally does. He wears protective pads and no helmet which makes no sense to me. Hopefully, he might appreciate me not discouraging his activity and instead showing support of it.

Over the course of a couple of days, I finished my shopping. There is a feeling of comfort that comes from being prepared and ready for Christmas. Knowing that nothing can interfere with having this job done satisfactorily is a relief. I am learning slowly that everything does work out, and *no* amount of worrying about it helps. There is one more job and then I really have kept to what we normally do. It is the annual holiday letter we will send out. I will give this one much consideration before it is tackled on another day.

John asked me what I would like for Christmas this year. I always tell him something small, or I help by picking out something I want. This year I was considerably bolder. I told him I was thinking about buying a reasonably priced laptop computer.

I explained that using the family computer intimidates me. I always seem to encounter problems. I fear doing something that will wreak havoc and cause everyone problems. It is frustrating, and *I* am sure not to want any connection to a mess I am totally responsible for creating. This is my computer anxiety issue; this is why I don't e-mail or look up anything on the Internet like real people do. Oh, the embarrassment and utter disgrace!

John listened as I made an argument for my unusual request. Explaining how much journaling has helped me I pointed to the pitfalls of handwriting this effort. Often I want to insert things or amend how I want to say something. It occurred to me that I might share this journal with my family. I am thinking they might be surprised and gratified to know how much their efforts have really helped me. The permanence of detailing this experience is appealing and it makes certain that events and feelings will not be changed or forgotten. John was interested in the opportunity to get me using a computer and wanted to encourage me. He also thinks it will give me more privacy, which I had not thought about.

This is an extravagant present considering our plan to have a more frugal holiday. It does seem selfish and indulgent. I kidded John by saying, "It would make up for the birthday present I did not get this year." He laughed. Hey, if I ever deserved a special gift, I'm pretty sure I earned it this year. What good is going through this, unless you can use it to some advantage? I *am* joking of course. Since I have never learned to type transposing this journal will be a huge job for me. My hunt-and-peck typing is poor at best. We will see if Santa thinks I have been "nice."

It is time for my last holiday task. Every year I send out a Christmas letter. Yes, one of those letters that most people don't want to read about *your* family. I have been creating these for about twenty years. My intentions are to fill people in on some memorable events from the past year and share the sentiments of the holidays. I send them to those people who we don't see through the year, those who may have a special interest in what is in this year's news, or to those who truly want my letter. There is an effort on my part to be silly, upbeat, sentimental and democratic in what I include. Someday, I will collect all of these and make a little book for our children as keepsakes.

I write the letter and then John tweaks it. He corrects my creative and often incorrect grammar. This is where his parochial education really pays off. I am better about content and flow. Well, that is my opinion. Actually John is an excellent writer, but he tends to include even more details if unrestrained. This year my letter will be particularly challenging as I do not want it to be a "Christmas bummer."

The big events of our year had to be covered without being depressing. It was a year of crisis, but as always there were wonderful memories too. I was satisfied with my finished draft. John had taken the time to offer a few corrections and we accomplished this task pretty handily. Keeping this letter going was my way of letting the recipients see I really am OK. Completing this tradition was a relief.

Monday, Vicki and I met for an early inside-mall walk. This has not become a steady routine. The weather and our schedules have made this difficult. The stores are opening earlier for holiday hours and that makes it more crowded with germs. Depending on Vicki's business obligations, time can also become an obstacle. We have missed the exercise and mental health boost walking had given us. Ginny has also been busy and we manage only to talk on the phone. It is a crazy time for everyone.

Wednesday, December 16, was my forth chemo treatment. Wow! This is the halfway mark with my chemo. These treatments have been as mild as the doctor and her nurses described months ago. I finally got past the cold that lasted a good two months. "Thankful" is the operative word.

Let me be clear that I am not fooling myself into believing everything is perfect either. I am simply recognizing that I am very fortunate; things could be much worse. Though I am determined to get past this ordeal and its challenges there are moments when it is tough.

Admittedly as I have mentioned before, I'm the original glass-half-empty girl. As a high school senior my yearbook favorite quote read: "To dry one's eyes, laugh at a fall and baffled get up and begin again" (Unknown Author). That struck a chord with me way back even then. I truly believe attitude makes a tremendous difference in how we handle things and what we accomplish. I know it is important for me to stay strong and be positive about whatever I can be, whenever possible. But I can't be rosy all the time, either.

Today's treatment was uneventful and routine. It had taken longer to have the chemo as I had to check with my insurance company about ordering more injections. They are very expensive, and I wanted to be sure I had the authorization for additional ones to be ordered. All was fine and we proceeded. The chemo center was backed up so we grabbed our usual lunch in between the doctor appointment and the chemotherapy today. We were home by mid-afternoon. I was looking forward to the high school holiday concert that evening. It is always special and a great start to our holiday season.

After chemo it is most important to hydrate. This afternoon I made less of an effort because I knew I would be more comfortable at school this evening. I will try and make up for it when we get home later this evening. It will be the first time I set foot in school this year. We always thoroughly enjoy this event, which is filled with an eclectic selection of music. It was a treat I would not easily miss. We used to watch and listen to Keith play in the concert and jazz bands. Now it is Cara's turn in the chorus. It is a nice way of running into many town acquaintances and exchanging good wishes. Grandma and Grandpa always join us and they get a kick out of it, too. Of course they think the bands are missing Keith's contribution. No prejudice there.

It was not as easy to relax as I was headachy and tired at its end. This was the ninth consecutive holiday concert we have attended and I was still glad to attend.

The next morning I awakened with a headache, a sensitive tongue and a bad stomach. Perhaps, the lack of hydration for hours yesterday was a mistake. First I used the special mouthwash and then I took a pill to help my stomach. I have taken only a few of the pills that I was given at the start of my treatments. I quickly felt better. I used some of the next-day energy the steroids provide and got some housework done. By afternoon I was tired and working only on more hydration. I found myself looking to eat more "junk" than I have let myself do lately. It was a sign that I am tired and looking for that extra energy you expect will come from sugar.

When Cara came home from school she found a little gift inside our mailbox. It had my name on it. How exciting! It was left by our sweet neighbor Dee. This was a beautiful, silver "friend" Christmas ornament. I hung it on our tree immediately. Dee often has colds throughout the school year, due to her work as a daycare exercise instructor; she understands my germ phobia and keeps her distance.

My neighbors are very considerate. Even Loretta, who invited us to her Christmas party, told me to think about not attending. It was funny to be uninvited because she thought the germ-factor too risky. I was glad to be let off the hook. My neighbor has been so kind in helping me out, and I had not wanted to insult her. She is a gem.

Christmas is only a week away. I spoke with Ginny who is sick. I was thinking of spending some time with her, but now I'm glad that we haven't been together. I hope she will be well enough to really enjoy the holidays. Eventually we will see one another, but probably not until later in January.

We have decided to arrange for Garry to be transported by a special vehicle to our home on Christmas. This will make the day much better for all of us. I am expecting my Mom and Irwin and Vicki, Paul and Jennifer to come for a holiday meal and spend the day. That is a small holiday group for us. Some years John's family also joins us; this year they all have plans elsewhere. This is a very comfortable plan.

Normally, we get together on another day with my Aunt Betty, her sons and their families. They also understand that our present concerns regarding Garry and me prohibit our getting together. My cousin's wife Carol mentioned that one of her boys has a slight cold. That was enough to make me feel better about canceling the yearly gathering. She mentioned that she had sent presents by mail and that she found something she hoped we would especially enjoy. She thought that at least John would be happy with what was coming. That left a bit of a mystery and we all awaited the surprise.

A couple of days later Carol's gift arrived. It was the complete collection of the Beatles music. It was an impressive collector's treasure. We *all* love their music and this was exciting! In fact, it was *I* who actually saw the Beatles perform live at Shea Stadium in the summer of 1965. This is a fact that I often pull out to really impress people; unfortunately it lets everyone know how old I am. I was there with a group of girls including my friend Colette. So while John and Keith may be the musicians in our family and my daughters both love the old music from this group it was also a perfect gift for me. I told Carol about that and she was thrilled with her selection being such a "hit" with us all. This was an exceptional and "very cool" gift!

Christmas Eve was a different affair this year. Anne was determined to help out with preparations. This was something new. She had spent the last few years splitting the holiday with her former boyfriend's family and ours. She never really got into any holiday hosting duties at all. I was surprised and decided to welcome her help.

Cara decided to be a part of what we were doing, too. More helping hands meant this was going to be a real family effort. How nice for me! They had always been asked to clean their bedrooms and help with various other cleaning jobs in preparation for company in the past. This was great. They helped make pumpkin pies, mashed potatoes and stuffing ahead of time.

My Mom was bringing her famous appetizer, meatballs in beer. Vicki and Jen were making a big spinach salad, hummus and buying more dessert. I suspected my brother-in-law Paul would actually be doing a large amount of purchasing. John and Keith would make shrimp cocktail Christmas morning. I needed only make the vegetables and turkey that day.

This was so much easier than most other holidays. We actually enjoyed preparing all the foods ahead of time together. It allowed me to get better prepared for the next day. Tablecloths were ironed and placed on the tables. I set the dining room table and carefully planned the next day's schedule. Everything was just right.

Christmas morning the five of us were more relaxed and happier with each other then on some holiday mornings. The spirit of cooperation seemed to continue. We all gathered first in the living room and we distributed presents anxiously. Keith and Cara always seem to be in the greatest hurry. Anne is pretty calm and always happy to give us gifts. John acts moderately interested, but we all know he enjoys receiving presents. I must wait; watching as my gifts for all of them are opened first. Every gift selection that meets with approval makes me more pleased. This year they were all hits. Well, I am not sure . . . John might have thought the helmet was goofy, I couldn't be certain.

When I opened my present I was happy to find my Christmas wish had been granted!

Cara knew I had been keeping a journal, and that I was contemplating transposing it to the computer. Keith was in on the shopping for it, and he also had an idea what it was about. Anne was seldom at home and remained in the dark as to my plans. Finally Anne couldn't hold back, "Mommy does not even use the computer. Mom does not need her own laptop, I might need one, but what is she going to do with it?"

Because Anne and Keith are adopted and Cara is our biological child they often kid one another frequently about their status within the family.

Cara quickly came at her with an answer, "Mom is starting a website called: www.sellyouradoptedkids.com" This was sweet revenge for all the, "You're the *real* child" and "she's the bad seed" jokes that have been thrown in Cara's direction by her older siblings. We all got hysterical laughing as Anne smiled but remained confused. We explained my project and they all responded with a collective, "Go for it, that's great!"

We placed our gifts back under the tree and did our Christmas breakfast fairly leisurely. We continued the tasks of the day working on last-minute details. We were in unusually good shape. Everything was fine until the rest of the family arrived.

Grandma and Grandpa were a wreck. They anticipated all kinds of issues with Garry. My mother was obviously upset and nervous. Vicki arrived in a panic as well. I snapped that everyone was making problems and it looked like trouble ahead.

Garry entered the house from his secured ride with little or no difficulty. The driver had locked the wheelchair in the vehicle and Garry was never moved off his chair. My brother was impressed with the condition and the amenities of the vehicle and seemed happy enough about the transport. After a while the rest of us settled down for a pleasant day. Actually it went as well as possible. It was disturbing to see Garry's deteriorated condition. When it was time for his driver to pick him up to go home my brother seemed tired and ready to leave us. I don't think he ever thought he might *not* be here with us today.

Garry left with all the men and Anne helping him to the van. Watching how easily the driver got the wheelchair in and out of his vehicle relieved us all. The driver smiled and said my brother remarked to him earlier, "You're probably a good looking guy, but you *should* consider a shave." I think the driver could tell that Garry was a special person and he was very good with him, which made us more comfortable.

When Garry left and was outside my mom started to cry. It took a little while but we managed to enjoy the rest of the holiday. It was a difficult, but good day. We couldn't expect more than this. Gratefully, we were all together. None of us understood what was happening to Garry, but it was terribly sad. We had done our best today and being here had made him happy. This was likely the last time my brother would come to our home and already it felt as though something was terribly wrong.

Naturally, everyone ate way too much as always. This Christmas Day was over.

OUT WITH THE OLD, IN WITH THE NEW

We had a relatively quiet holiday season as planned. It was better than I would have thought possible and that made me happy.

Our children continue to do their own "things." Keith has been on a long vacation break. He has been at home more than usual, which we enjoy. John and Keith have been watching tons of football and other miscellaneous alpha-male sports. They love the bloody war and horror movies and the most asinine-comedy programs. Yes, having Keith around is a welcome difference to the usual female drama for John.

Anne has mostly been staying out. She and Keith seemed to be on each other's nerves. It makes me uncomfortable and I hope this is temporary. We have been fortunate that all three children are almost always great together. The main issue seems to be about the cars in driveway. My suspicion is there is something else going on. John keeps reminding me not to worry. Perhaps Anne is looking for a reason to stay out. Ah, that could be it.

Cara is in and out constantly. The movies, shopping and being with friends keep her busy enough. However, everyone managed to be home for Aunt Mary and Uncle Bob's after-Christmas visit. It extended the holiday a little and was nice to be with them.

New Years Eve was quiet. Anne slept at her friend's, Keith spent most of the night at the computer and Cara was out. Vicki was not up for coming out in bad weather. It was just another quiet night. We said goodbye to 2009 without celebration or fanfare. It had been a tough year! We were wishing for a better 2010 for everyone.

My fifth treatment on January 6, I got a break—the doctor did not weigh me this time. I knew it would be evidence of the excessive eating I had done and I was not looking to own-up to it. The chemo went off without a hitch. It is all very much a routine at this point. The mid-cycle injections are worse than the chemo. The bone and muscle aches are annoying at best. I'm anxious to complete these treatments. It is not because of the side effects, or any difficulty with having the actual procedure done; it is strictly about the time element. I need to have this behind me.

I have wanted to find a new job and with all these appointments getting one now is impossible. If I was already working at a job they would likely work around these commitments, but who would want to hire me with all these interruptions. Making me even less marketable!

While I remind myself that I have been very lucky, I still have another surgery to look forward to. It's a bit unnerving to realize this whole business will be longer than I imagined.

My new computer-notebook project was waiting for me to become brave enough to sit down and get started. Keith was interested and willing to help instruct me; he was the ideal person for such a project. Finally, I sat and listened to him while he offered various instructions and key pieces of advice. I was ready. It was good timing as I have just about used up the pages in the journal that Laura gifted me with months before.

My mission will be to clean up the contents of my journal. My concern is that upon rereading it, this will all seem to be less important to preserve. It was slow and frustrating that I am not into any technology. Not being a typist to begin with makes this more difficult. Transposing the original journal to my new laptop has become my new obsession and goal. I am psyched about this adventure!

Uncle Tom and Aunt Barbara were not able to come over for the holidays as my brother-in-law was nursing a bad cold. We did not get together with them until John's birthday on January 14. That turned out perfectly. I planned a terrific meal and birthday cake. My gift to John was a new winter casual coat. He wanted one very similar to his old one. I thought I found just the right one. The children had tickets for their Dad and them to see the movie "Avatar" on Sunday. Keith was going back to Rutgers on Saturday; and I was still avoiding theaters. John was thrilled about their gift as he wanted to see this movie.

This turned out well to share the birthday with John's brother and Barbara. They lucked out as it was one of my better meals. I was glad too, because Keith was still home to join us. The Christmas tree was left up longer than usual, which went along with them giving the children some holiday gifts. Everyone seemed content.

Saturday John and I planned to take our son back to school. Keith offered to pack up the Christmas tree and put it away in the attic before he left. I quickly undressed the tree and left the ornaments to be boxed carefully later. This was very helpful and afterward we drove him back to school. We missed him almost immediately.

Sunday, Cara had a problem finishing a group project she was involved in for school. I ended up going to the movie with John and Anne instead of her. She was disappointed, but this was the best solution. Afterward, we scooped Cara up at home and went for a rare family dinner out. This was a treat and the girls were delighted to be in on this part of the day. It was a good way to end John's birthday.

—॥॥—

A few days ago, Garry told me that he is quite scared about what he would find out at his appointment next week. This is an unusual statement for him. My mother was particularly worried too, that he might be moved out of his group home because of the additional care needed. It was comforting knowing Vicki was going to be with them. I would get more complete information from my sister and I was interested in hearing what the doctor had to say.

My sister met Mom, Irwin and Garry on the appointment Monday morning. This appointment was with a neurologist. After further testing it was determined that there was evidence of nerve damage in Garry's brain. The doctor explained that Garry has PLS, a slower form of the disease ALS. This devastating illness attacks the nerves which then cannot send messages to the brain for the muscles; eventually all the muscles stop working. The doctor impressed them with his interest and compassion toward Garry and about his condition.

My brother is relieved to hear that he does not have a brain tumor, which apparently is what he expected. This strikes him to be better news. He is also more comfortable that it is not related to his CP. He has been angry because he had been unaware that he was born with that issue and seemed to feel we had intentionally hidden it from him. This was not the case. He always had coordination issues, however, they seemed insignificant to us. Perhaps now, Garry had less to be angry with us about. The rest of us were thinking, *This, was not the news we wanted to hear!* There will be a little more testing, but there is no cure. He doesn't understand how serious this information is.

My Mom was relieved with the fact that the social worker and Garry's manager were sincerely working on his behalf; she felt more secure for now. This is all so unbelievable! This guy deserves a miracle. Words are really inadequate at this point. I spoke with Garry later and he said, "I wouldn't wish this on anyone." I know he had been comforted by all the support today.

My sister-in-law Mary called with news that she is having a health issue of her own. Her situation is manageable, but it is now added to our growing list of concerns. I know she was considerately trying not to have us worried about her until after the holidays. I am glad she let us know about what is going on.

A week or so later, John's brother Tom called to inform us that his wife was to have a hernia operation. We expect this will be done fairly easily. It seemed like: Out with the old and in with the new . . . problems. Optimism was the direction we wanted to maintain and that continues to be "the plan."

MAKING CONNECTIONS

Loretta, the saint, came by this week for my next round of injections. She and I continue to get to know each other. She could not be nicer about this favor. My neighbor constantly reassures me that it is not a problem to add me to her usually busy schedule. How fortunate am I?

This round of shots was the roughest so far. It brought on headaches and jaw aches at first. As the week progressed the general bone and muscle pain got worse. My tongue broke out in sores again, which was easily fixed by using the magic mouthwash. The other aches and pains lasted longer this time. I was starting to really be uncomfortable. In fact, I was convincing myself that I might be starting to have other issues because of constant pain on the sides of my lower back. I will to speak to my doctor at the next chemo appointment about this.

We received some nice responses to our holiday correspondence. We heard from our Texas friend, John's college roommate, who we have seen a handful of special times throughout the years. Our friend Carol also sent a letter and that always picks me up. There have been other nice, late cards and notes. Our holiday news touched some people who had not planned to send anything out this year and changed their minds.

John's other college buddy also wrote to us. His year was also difficult. Bruce told us that he lost his younger sister and his nephew this year. One was a result of an illness and the other was from an accident. How tragic this was, and we were grateful he shared this with us. There were a couple of people I would have liked to have heard from. After this letter I thought, *What kind of year must they be having?* Maybe I should continue to reach out to these people to make sure they are OK.

This morning Mary needed me for a ride home from a medical appointment. It was nice to help someone else for a change. Afterward, we made an essential trip to the diner for breakfast. I have not seen her much lately and I was glad to spend some time together. She seems to be in a positive frame of mind and determined to handle her medical crisis.

My childhood friend Colette sent me a note with three books that she thought I might like to read. As the time passes, I am hearing from most people less. They know I am doing well. So, this was a pleasant and unexpected gift. Our encounters have been amicable, but we never make plans to get together. Of course, her mom's moving away last year meant we were less likely to run into each other. After the four or five letters we have exchanged, it might be more personal to speak with her this time and I am thinking of giving her a call. Maybe now would be an appropriate time to reconnect again.

Laura planned a "tea luncheon" for Ginny and me this week. Our other friend from high school, Jane, happened to call me to say Laura had kept her informed about me. I was delighted to hear from her.

Laura, Jane and I had children born within two weeks of each other when Anne was a baby. For the first five years we steadily had play-dates together. It had been wonderful to share that period of time with these women. Laura and I were first-time older moms. Jane was the experienced mom, this being her third child, and though the youngest of our group she was our role model. We had a great many laughs throughout those years. As the children got busy with their own lives, our visits became less frequent. We got together once in a while without the three children. Eventually I saw less of Jane. Laura and I have been friends even longer and thankfully, we are mindful of remaining in touch regularly.

Jane was able to arrange her schedule to join us. She has grandchildren whom she helps out with much of the time. This seems to suit her. Laura was a great hostess. She is very into this "tea" idea. Her table and treats were amazing and delicious. Too delicious! The hours flew by and we had the best time. Good friends, good eats and lots of fun!

Several days later, I decided to call Colette. She seemed surprised and pleased. We talked non-stop for a good hour-and-a-half. This was a big step toward us reconnecting. It was quite pleasant and it ended with us picking a date to meet for breakfast to celebrate her birthday at the end of February. I am looking forward to this meeting. She mentioned that her mom's 88th birthday is in a few days; I will send Etta a card.

I just sent off some thank you notes to Laura and Jane (for a silver keychain with an "A" on it) for their gestures last week. Also, I sent my friend Carol an update. They have been so supportive and I want them to know this is not taken for granted. This health scare has made me a much more "mushy" person. That is not so terrible, right? I also sent cards with notes to John's college buddy, who told us of his losses and one for Colette's mom, too.

Vicki was thanked in a different way. She had mentioned her love of chili and I knew exactly what to do. I had a tasty recipe for turkey chili. I made her a large batch frozen in small containers to be used as desired. That was a big success and then I did the same with my recipe for vegetable bean stew. Both were hits and more appreciated than I expected and I felt pretty good about this. Life is about reaching out to others and it can be accomplished in lots of ways. *When your heart is in the right place you just cannot lose.*

Keith has not been home much this school year. However, his random text messages keep me from worrying too much and often brighten my day. Sometimes they are as short as "luv u." He is a character. I will ask questions and he minimally replies with great skill. Today I received a long phone call about how much he is enjoying his classes. He was enthusiastic and it made me happy to hear from him. He has matured this year and conversations are much more substantial. He was also letting me know that he is committed to getting back in shape and returning to rugby soon. The latter is not such good news for the worrying-me.

Laura sent me pictures from her luncheon. It shocked me a bit to see myself with my friends. It was obvious to me that I looked worn out. My friends had complimented me on how well I looked that day. I think what they meant was, all things considered I looked well. That will have to be enough and I greatly appreciate their kindnesses.

I am not feeling ill from the chemo and that allows me to keep going. Perhaps I have not been totally realistic either. After all, I have had five treatments already and I suppose they are taking some toll on me.

MEETING CHALLENGES

I t was February 17, the sixth chemo treatment. As Vicki and I drove in to the city I told her about my issues concerning pains above my hips. My sister was prepared to remind me to express this new information to my oncologist.

My recent two blood workups were indicating my sugar level was higher than it should be. I was quick to point out that these tests were done immediately following both Thanksgiving weekend and then again after Christmas week. My doctor did not appreciate the excuse or this line of defense.

We decided that I should make better effort in my diet; then we would take another look at this in a couple of weeks. Sweets are a downfall of mine. This did not make me happy, but I knew she was correct in her instructions to me. Vicki was certainly not surprised and made her thoughts on this quite clear. I will be more careful as the thought of a new medical concern or additional medication is unappealing. My doctor ordered more blood work for tests next week. Also they will do a more specific screening for diabetes.

We talked about the concern of *mine* that I may have a kidney issue. The doctor smiled as I showed her the area of my pain. She responded clinically with the information that the kidneys are actually in a higher location. I felt silly and ignorant about my body. She was understanding and continued to explain how the injections work. They promote the production of white cells in the blood, which affects the bone marrow. This area is where about forty-percent of this occurs; it made perfect sense and explained my discomfort. It relieved me to have this knowledge.

The doctor thinks I may be hypersensitive to the injections. Since they are providing the desired results she wants me to continue with taking them. We decided on four shots in the next round and we will see how I do with this new routine. Basically, I will do whatever is needed to complete these treatments as soon as possible. I anticipate my chemotherapy will be finished up early in March.

As usual Vicki and I stepped across the street for our lunch. This was the first time it was a problem for me. Something was just not right, and I forced myself to have a taste and then left the rest behind. I definitely was feeling a little bit off for the rest of this day.

There has been some noticeable difference in my hair recently; it is thinning slightly. My family tells me that they cannot see much difference. I won't get upset by this condition. When I had been on medication for a thyroid problem a few years ago, I experienced a similar loss. This is temporary. I have noticed that my hair's growth has slowed down considerably since treatments began. That helps as I have had less need to color my hair as a result. The doctor's staff suggested that I use a natural vegetable-based dye. It does not contain several ingredients which presently would damage my hair. It happens that I like the product and it does seem safer.

—❦—

My laptop is super and it is keeping me busy. It is horrifying to admit how sloppily I wrote in my journal. It is filled in with bad handwriting and lots of spelling and grammar mistakes. It now occurs to me to include background details to explain more clearly who I was at the beginning of this breast cancer journey. I thought my children might particularly enjoy reading about that. Anyway, there I was merrily plugging along typing one day and . . . oops!

All of a sudden, I don't remember what I did, but almost the entire day's efforts disappeared. A blink and it was gone! Keith had told me to call him with any problems. Unfortunately, I touched a key or two first. It was all gone! It sent me into a traumatic state. After a minute I called Keith. He was very sympathetic and tried everything to help me retrieve my work. Nothing worked. He said I must have deleted something first, and then told the computer to "save the delete." I lost that whole new portion of today's document.

He then also re-explained how to go back to before that error occurred for the next time. It is called "Undo." Yikes! Of course, he had told me this before and I just had not remembered what to do. Oh, the agony of being untechno-savvy! I am severely challenged to the point where I may be technology-unfriendly and incompatible. I was upset and determined to "get back in the saddle." Tomorrow, I would have to rewrite these missing pages. My family shared my pain as best they could and they encouraged me to simply continue on.

The days go by and John has become a journal-widower as my project thrives. It might be a way of getting him back for the guitar playing time I have put up with through the years. He is actually being very understanding and tells me he thinks it is a healthy endeavor.

WINTER CONTINUES

We settled into our quiet winter routine. John had a particularly crazy work week and came home from his sixth day at the office. He was dying to break out and do something. We decided to call friends in town, Maryann and Tony. They have come by to visit a couple of times recently. John and Tony are silly together, and Maryann and I console each other regarding this and other life-mysteries. They also were in need of time to relax.

Next I called Vicki and Paul to see if they wanted to meet the four of us at a restaurant. They were delighted to do so. This turned out to be a comfortable combination of personalities. It was light and pleasant and we were all pleased for this spontaneous evening.

The following week was uneventful and quiet. Fortunately Vicki and I got to get back into a fairly good walking pattern. I'm feeling pretty good.

Saturday afternoon I called Ginny at the last minute. Bad weather cancelled plans that they had made earlier. John and I ended up crashing on them for a card game of Hearts. John and Greg played in college. Every once in a while we fall back on that activity to pass the time. Ginny and I are no card sharks. We were happy to spend time together, as we never seem to do it often enough. They are much more socially connected people with all kinds of things filling their calendar. It is always fun to see them. I am hoping that when the weather gets much better Ginny and I will do some more walking outside.

Super Bowl Sunday came. We have hosted a small party for game day the last few years. I was not interested this time. Mary and Bob would have come but she is on a miserably severe diet. Garry couldn't come. Vicki and Paul were not into this game and with no New York team involved they were exceptionally disinterested. Mom and Irwin would have come, but my mom has no patience or interest in sports. Keith was at school and the girls were not fans anyway. It just didn't seem like much of a party.

Instead I decided to ask our friend Dan to join us for a simple meal and the game. He has had a difficult year being recently separated from his wife, and also losing his mom. He has been consumed in tying up all those "loose ends." We were glad to have him come by. To all our surprise, it was around midnight before we said goodnight.

Tuesday John stayed at home to deal with the big storm here. I couldn't shovel this large amount of snow comfortably. We have a substantial snow blower; however, it is not something I can handle using. In the past, I have done my share of the good old-fashioned pick-up-and-toss. Even this winter I had handled the smaller jobs. It was a relief John stayed home and I was grateful for his help. It was nice not having to worry about him traveling to and from work. John was "The Man" and all the neighbors were delighted to have his help, too. Before the day was over he cleared four driveways.

On February 9, I called Loretta and insisted that I walk over to her for this round of shots. She does not feel steady on snow and ice. I was happy to give her some consideration for once. By the time I stepped outside there was a least twelve inches of fresh snow. It was a winter wonderland and I loved being in it for a few moments. The fresh snow lighted the street, the air was crisp and with the evening's silence, it all felt perfect.

When John came inside I knew he had worked too hard. He crashed about 7:30 and slept for hours before awakening again. I was watching a movie. As he couldn't return to sleep for a while he joined me.

The rest of the shots were at Loretta's house this week. I am hoping the four injections will be sufficient. It seems as though the side effects are better this time. I have been achy but not like the last time. Thank goodness for this.

Cara has been working hard on this year's school play, a production of "A Wonderful Town." Practices are getting more intense as the play is at the end of this month. The dedication on everyone's part is admirable. It always seems like they are not going to be ready and then, like magic it all works terrifically. Some nights she is at school until 9:00 or 10:00. By the time it is over, we will all be exhausted.

There are several changes in the cast and their roles within the scheduled six performances. In addition, there is one understudy dress rehearsal when we can see Cara in her largest role. We enjoy catching most of the shows, which allows us to see the production in different ways.

It is gratifying to watch our daughter as she continues to cultivate her theater interest. It does produce a bit of parent-anxiety at the same time. Cara wants to be "perfect" and we want her to have fun, no matter what happens. So far, this involvement has been very positive. We are very excited and even my germ phobia is not going to stop my attendance.

My sister, mom and Irwin met Garry at his second meeting with his neurologist today. The doctor wants to start Botox injections in his legs. This *may* unfreeze some muscles and make him more comfortable for a while. The doctor added a vitamin supplement to Garry's diet, but did not think it would cause any great results. This meeting was shorter than the first one was. It would seem that there is little more that can be offered. This is discouraging. Garry called me later on and seemed resigned to having the injections. His mood was fairly good, all things considered. He is a trouper.

Vicki and I had a poor week in terms of meeting for walking. There were weather issues in particular on Tuesday, which canceled a day of walking at the mall. My bone-pain issues also interfered, and Vicki had the early appointment with Garry's doctor visit on another morning. We will try again next week. I did run into Jane when Vicki and I walked once earlier in the week. It was funny to see each other so soon. She is going to send me some pictures from our "tea" day at Laura's. She is a doll. We sat down for a little talk in the mall before saying goodbye.

The weekend was quiet. John and I ran out for a bite to eat at the diner late on Saturday. We were alone and it struck us as preferable to defrosting dinner from the freezer. It was fine except that there were three people who had terrible coughs around the diner. I became overly aware of them and was glad to come home to get away from the general public again. We picked Cara up from her friend's house as we were out anyway. It was so cold and I appreciated her understanding that we were being economical in our trips outside this night. She had a long day at theater-practice before hanging out with her friends and easily agreed.

Today is Valentine's Day, February 14. Everyone got a little something as is my custom. John got a DVD of *"Midnight Cowboy,"* the movie we saw on our first date almost forty years ago. Not particularly a first-date movie, it was rated "X," back then! Still I thought it was a romantic idea. He seemed to "get it" and we will watch it together soon.

Today, John is working desperately to fix the family computer which has been a problem for a long time. He is frustrated and is working on it with assistance from people from foreign lands on the phone. This has taken all day and night and there are still issues he is not satisfied about. Oy.

I have been working on various things around the house and on my journal. Randomly we are catching a little of the Olympics on TV. Not so romantic. Cara and her friends are at the movies and I am waiting to get a call to pick them up. All is well.

When I picked up Cara and her pals I became suspicious that a couple of them were coming down with colds. Not realizing that they seemed to be getting sick, Cara apologized to me for this added concern. I felt badly as I could see that she was now uncomfortable. She asked me how I could tell they were getting sick. Well, I guess it's my new gift, or perhaps I am being paranoid. Actually, their sniffles and husky voices gave me reason to take notice. This group also has to worry about their health with the play less than two weeks away. Colds and flu are typically play-time issues.

—∭—

With a good deal of pride, I am happy to report that after diligently working on my journal I have completed transposing it into my notebook. Yay! Corrections will be much easier to handle on the computer. It was a task for me to do all the typing required to make this conversion. I am no longer going back and forth writing about the most current, and then returning to transposing the original material a little at a time. Reevaluating what I had handwritten provided me the opportunity to make important additions to details and modifications in how I expressed myself. I never expected to enjoy this so much.

Today is President's Day and a school holiday. Cara still needed to be at school from 10:00 to 7:00 for theater practice. We awakened to some light snow. The play is getting closer and we understand the importance of extra practices. Cara's friend text messaged her that she was getting a ride separately because she has a cold. That was very considerate and I appreciated both of them being aware of and responsive to my concerns.

Vicki and I chose to cancel our morning walk because the snow was getting heavier. Neither of us is much for bad-weather driving. The snow came down for the next four or five hours and then continued in a fine constant fall. I began to worry about leaving my driveway to pick Cara up later at school. John and Anne were at work. There was about six inches of accumulation of light-powdery snow, and no reason why I should not clear off the steps and walk.

It was not my intention to do more shoveling than I could handle comfortably, but before long I was tackling the driveway. The weather report said that the temperature would drop after 5:00, and I wanted to help before it froze. John had been doing so much extra work including repairing our family computer, which was still incomplete. It brought me satisfaction to make this contribution to the list of things that needed to be done.

This was something that I've always done in the past. Of course, I probably did overdo it. However, I was feeling impressed with myself. After all, it was only six months ago that I had my double mastectomy. Add being three quarters through with chemotherapy and it is pretty amazing that I spent a couple of hours shoveling snow.

I enjoyed the activity for the most part and it was great to be outdoors. I also cleaned off the two cars in the driveway before I realized that I had had enough. In the meantime John had called and I told him my assessment of the weather and road conditions. He suggested that I should leave the snow for him later on and reminded me to use good judgment. I was comfortable knowing that it would be easier for me to get in and out to pick up Cara whenever she called. I felt fine.

Later, Anne picked Cara up in her truck anyway. She had stepped in the house from work just as the call came and offered to get her sister. I was making dinner and honestly, I was exhausted. It was perfect timing and I appreciated the favor. John came home to a minor snow removal of the rest of the day's accumulation. It seemed as though tomorrow's forecast would be OK for Vicki and I to go in for chemo number seven, February 17.

In the morning, Vicki skipped stopping for her special tea because she was concerned about being late. The roads were still icy from yesterday and she decided to come straight over. We arrived early enough to walk a block down the street to pick up her favorite concoction before my appointment. It has become equally important to me that she gets this essential requirement for her day's comfort. She loves her Tazo Chai Tea! Mine remains a simple order: coffee, milk, no sugar (only once in a while), but not from this same shop. We are sisters and we love each other immensely, but we are very different. No problem here.

We were early and had my bloodwork done first. We waited briefly to see my doctor and then waited a short time to have my treatment. The doctor was happy that I was doing well and we talked about having only one more chemotherapy to go after today. My blood count was good and we decided a similar course of injections before the last treatment was appropriate. In addition the doctor also wants me to take one last round of injections ten days after the last chemo; they will help keep my white cell count from getting too depleted. As this has been so successful I'm fine with the plan.

I am also determined to enjoy Cara's play coming up next weekend. I think the injections will help see me through that exposure to the crowd's germs. Keeping healthy and attending these performances are extremely important to me. All this will work.

Vicki and I spoke with two women in the waiting room. One charming woman told us she was coming for treatments weekly for over nine years. She had breast cancer and then it spread into her lungs. She was a vibrant woman and seemed to have a wonderful attitude. Another woman there was not specific about her situation; she was a patient for eleven years. Wearing a kerchief on her head, she was having a treatment today. I realize now how varied these experiences actually are. It also explains why so many patients seem familiar with one another. They have seen each other far too frequently with the passage of time. Both these women had the same doctor and their appointments were seriously behind schedule.

Vicki told these patients, "I want you to know that I am a twenty-three year survivor." They seemed very impressed and encouraged with this information. We were called to start my treatment, and we all wished each other to be well. I was relieved that *my* doctor was having a better time handling her day. We were pleasantly surprised how smoothly our routine went.

This was the first time that I had my favorite nurse Ann since my second treatment day. What a gentle personality she has. We talked about the Yankees and I reminded her that spring practice starts today for pitchers and catchers. She had to explain that the hospital has made one change in my treatment. The three anti-nausea pills are being replaced with a new medication which is administered in the IV before my chemo started. This may have less of a headache side effect. The time went by quickly. Ann asked me how I was doing and we discussed my mild experience thus far. I told her about my mouth issues, my super-dry lips and fingertips, occasional bone and muscle issues from the injections and my recent hair thinning. I told her that I felt unusually tired at the end of the day, and she assured me that this is all typical toward the last couple of treatments.

Ann made me feel very comfortable, and we agreed that I have managed well throughout this therapy. I thanked and complimented her; she was special, and I did not know if I'd see her again.

We were finished early and Vicki suggested a Mexican restaurant back in New Jersey not far from home. Guacamole sounded excellent, so we went there for lunch. We also shared a plate of salmon and refried beans and rice. Yummy. We had a leisurely meal and relaxed. Possibly, our frequent adventures into the city will be missed. Vicki commented, "We will have to find other reasons to continue to spend time together and have some better times." That sounded real good to me.

I cannot believe my last chemotherapy treatment is only three weeks away! Last night I was a bit tired, but I was also busy and did not fall asleep early as I might have expected. In fact we went to sleep very late, and I had a slight headache probably due to that. I woke up and took Cara to school and then met Vicki at the mall to walk. I felt well and was glad to get the exercise fit into our day.

I did my errands: bank, post office, cleaners and food store. I probably had been working off the steroids from yesterday. Later, I became cranky from all kinds of little annoyances. Then I realized that my mouth was dry with a weird taste, and my stomach was feeling out of sorts. I tried to relax for a while.

This week's chemotherapy hit me differently than the first six treatments. It may be the accumulation of these drugs that are catching up with me. My anti-nausea medication was changed this time. Perhaps, my out-of-sorts stomach and unusual blahs are more a reaction to that difference; I am not sure. Last night I fell asleep while watching the Olympic skating events that I normally enjoy. John awakened me so that I could come to bed around 11:30, but by then I had slept quite a while. I fell back to sleep easily, and I did not get up until my sister called this morning at almost 9:00.

I am tired, but usually not able to get long sleeps anymore. This is due mostly to having had so many fluids causing me to use the bathroom frequently. Additionally if I sleep on my sides I will inevitably wake and straighten myself out to be on my back again. Last night was particularly tough. I was tired, but I told Vicki we could definitely meet at the mall in about a half-an-hour.

Funny, I guess my age has let me become more casual about things like running out without any makeup, not showering first, and throwing a hat on to hide my bed-head. Basically, I have no pride. It's the new me, improved or not. What's not so good is I do run into people. This morning I saw John's grammar-school buddy. He was very nice and we spent a few minutes talking. Next time, I will put on a little eye makeup and some lipstick to be a little more presentable. Oh dear!

The rest of the day was quiet. Anne came home on a long lunch break. She has been out so much that I finally got to give her the Valentine's gift. She was pleased with the thin sweater. Since she is always cold at work I thought maybe it could be worn under a blazer. Keith called me in the afternoon; he seems pretty busy and also happy. He is back on his diet and exercise program hoping to be ready in a few weeks to continue playing rugby. Cara is at play rehearsal until 10:00 tonight. Everyone is fine.

Garry called and we spoke for a few minutes. He is so sweet and always checking on how everyone here is doing. He liked the funny Valentine's card we sent him and wanted to thank the kids especially. I assumed he had other calls to make because he was brief.

All I accomplished today was a quick trip to the drug store to pick up some medication refills. Ginny called to see how I made out with this last treatment. We had a lengthy conversation. I'm unusually pooped. In a day or two, I will call my doctor to be sure this is to be expected. I really think I am OK. This is when I wish there was someone who has recently been through a similar experience that I could talk with. Generally, it seems to me that I do not want to make anyone else's experiences mine.

The weekend was quiet and centered on Cara's activities. She was involved with play rehearsals all weekend. Friday night and then Saturday until about 4:00 and even Sunday was filled with "the-play-is-only-one-week-away-craziness!" Cara also had a Sweet Sixteen party to attend on Saturday night. As busy as she was, that is how uneventful the weekend was for John and me.

Cara's friend's party was a huge success. Sunday, John insisted on us going for a walk outside in the afternoon. It was a good idea and I was glad he encouraged me to do so. It was still cold outside and slightly windy, but it felt like a hopeful sign that this winter will soon end. Walking outside feels like a healthier experience compared to the indoor-mall walks; I am definitely looking forward to more of this.

THE SHOW GOES ON

I t was my six-month checkup with the breast surgeon today, February 22nd. However, I did not see my doctor as she was out with a stomach virus. The office called and told me that I could come in and be examined by someone else today instead. Wanting to stick to my schedule I was confident that this presented no problem for me. Vicki and I went in and found that there was a small amount of patients in the office this morning. If I had been scheduled for a consult or some other significant meeting I would have postponed my appointment, too. Having been physically examined with each expansion and chemo appointment very carefully, I was comfortable that everything was just fine. The practitioner was personable and professionally pleased with how I was doing.

Vicki and I were pleasantly surprised that we were through and back to the car in approximately forty-five minutes. She had a busy work day shaping up and was off and running after she dropped me at home.

My sister-in-law Rita called me to see how I was doing. She had talked with John around their birthdays last month, but she and I had not spoken for a while. We talked quite a while and shared a few laughs about the kids mostly. She seemed happy that the information her friend, the oncology nurse, had given me months ago was accurate. I told Rita to relay my feelings to her friend and inform her treatments are almost over already.

After that I decided to call Colette. Tuesday's forecast for rain and possibly some snow could force her to rearrange her schedule to visit her mom in Pennsylvania. I thought our plans might need to be altered for meeting this Wednesday, but she would like to see what tomorrow brings first.

My friend is always anxious to share medical concerns having had some experiences of her own. It seems that people tend to want to share the details and the anxiety, which accompanies such events often and in depth. These situations can also have an overwhelming impact on you in regards to how vulnerable you feel afterward.

Well, I know what I need to do just in case I meet my old friend anytime soon—*color my hair, tonight!*

Later it seemed to be the right time to call my plastic surgeon's office to schedule my next surgery. My doctor told me to call after my last chemo was completed. He said that he needed two months past chemo before he could perform the surgery for the implant exchange. Knowing that my treatments have gone smoothly I felt that I could tell them that the last one is coming up; I am anxious to get on their surgery schedule. The person I spoke with was agreeable and did not hesitate to give me a date. Then I had to call the gynecologist to find out if the date worked for his schedule, too. Everything was set, both doctors were available and the remaining details will be arranged. Yay! My next surgery for both the implant exchange and the oophorectomy are set for May 7, 2010. I'm not surgery-happy, I am just very eager to wrap this whole business up.

It is a great relief to me that my next surgery does not conflict with Cara going to camp in June. She has been given a wonderful opportunity to attend a theater camp for three weeks. My cousin gifted her with this for Christmas. Their son attended this camp for years and enjoyed his time there very much.

This will be the first time Cara has been away other than an overnight arrangement. I am not totally comfortable with the idea that she will be gone for three weeks. I know this will be an incredibly valuable and positive experience and I am excited for her. With my surgery and recovery completed I will be able to take her to camp, which *I need to see*. The camp has an end of the session show. Now, there definitely won't be any conflict for that and I'm feeling much more comfortable already. Obviously, I am nervous about the whole idea—I still have time to deal with that problem.

Today was a bust. The weather was so ugly that Vicki and I decided not to meet at the mall. It continued to rain and sleet all day. Finally, I had to go out and do my errands. I waited until it was late enough so that I would go by the high school and pick Cara up at the same time. She had to get back for rehearsal tonight which will not end until 10:00. I wanted her to have as much time to do homework as possible and have dinner before she had to return.

Colette called and as I had expected needed to switch our plans to next Monday. Wow, my mom's birthday is on Tuesday and we will be deep into week two of Cara's play. Adding to that, it is my injections week also. I will be a crazy-busy lady all week.

This morning I took Cara to school and it was already snowing heavily. I managed a couple of local stops and headed right home. Mom and Irwin were also out and I became frantic because they did not even answer their cell phone. My concern was more that maybe there was a problem with Garry because I couldn't get him by phone, either. He had his Botox injections yesterday and I thought it odd that they were all out in this weather.

My mother called well into the morning to say they were doing their errands and her phone was on, but the ringer was not working. They are somewhat cell-phone challenged and this has presented some issues on different occasions. If I were to tell her that I was going out in this weather, she would be full of all kinds of cautions and warnings about not driving anywhere unnecessarily. Those warnings are not delivered with simple advice or gentle suggestions; they are stern promises of impending doom! This just may be where my own negative outlook springs from. Ah Ha! The apple does not fall far from the tree.

It also turned out that Garry went to work. The forecast predicted the bad weather to be later on in the day; they were all ignoring the obvious and early start. Garry and the other fellows he lives with were brought home early from work. It seems that I am getting a little more frantic than needed. One piece of good news is that Garry's injections have loosened the muscles in his legs so that he can bend them a bit. This is great. Perhaps his caregivers will be able to move them enough so that the swelling will subside to some extent. He seemed encouraged and upbeat regarding this small improvement. At least it was something positive.

The big storm started this morning and is still going strong. I did some shoveling earlier in the afternoon. This is that heavy, wet-mix with slush and snow. It was too much for me to do a lot of the job today. After cleaning the steps and walk and about a third of the driveway I gave up, not wanting to push my luck. Instinctively I felt it was enough work for now.

John is slowly making his way home. He actually called and said he could walk faster than he was driving on the highway to the George Washington Bridge. What a mess! Cara came home from school early as they were given a half-day dismissal.

We don't know whether there will be a performance tomorrow night yet. It will depend on when this storm ends and if they get to clean up for tomorrow night. The anxiety level is pretty high anyway this week concerning the play. It is exciting and totally nerve-racking all at once—oy, oy, oy!

John stayed home from work today due to the storm. It was helpful because I felt the shoveling I did yesterday was probably more than I should have attempted at this point. He was out early with our snow blower, and by the time he came back inside it was four or five hours later. A few neighbors joined him outside. They helped shovel steps and removed huge, icy piles left by the street plows and cleaned off cars. It was an enormous job and by the end of the morning, they had done five different houses.

At one point I saw sweet Dee outside serving chocolates to each of the men. I know *my* husband appreciated the thought. Oh yeah, he would work for a chocolate dropped into his mouth by this gal! Our snow blower, which we bought a couple of years ago, was important today. John was glad to help everyone out. I felt good too, as it seemed like a way to thank all of these people who have been so kind to us these past months. It looks as though we got at least fourteen inches already!

The show was canceled for this evening, February 26, and rescheduled for tomorrow afternoon. Cara seemed calm regarding all this. It is better that she did not get all bent out of shape over this uncontrollable circumstance. Now, there will be two shows tomorrow. The leads are having a practice at one of the cast member's home. Normally, I avoid driving in weather like we are having. My sister-in-law Mary called to let me know the local roads were fine. It appeared as though it would be manageable; so I dropped Cara off to rehearse for a while. It is probably wise to use this extra time to get better prepared for the play.

I am also taking advantage of this time and doing some extra cooking to get us through what is bound to be a wild couple of days. There is a show Sunday afternoon as well. So far we have tickets to see the afternoon show tomorrow for this weekend. We will see three or more performances before it is over. I cannot wait.

John, Anne, her boyfriend Dave and I went to the opening show performance Saturday afternoon. This performance replaced last night's cancelled show. It was a delight! The cast did a great job and the set design, orchestra, and lighting all worked equally well. Cara's role was that of the overbearing mother. Cara definitely made the most of every moment on stage. She spoke in a New York accent with a slight Jewish-mother feeling to it. She has a natural instinct for humor. She shines on stage. Of course all the other parents of the cast feel that their child is also pretty special on stage; imagine what the grandparents are thinking. We were so proud of our daughter! One indisputable fact was that Cara was very happy with the show.

Sunday afternoon the alternate cast had the matinee performance. I couldn't stand knowing that there was a show mid-afternoon and we decided to run over to see an extra show. This was Cara's performance where she is a part of the ensemble. She had a few lines, which were quite funny though brief. She also likes this part as there is little pressure and she is *not* made up like an old-frumpy woman. We enjoyed this show, too. You have got to give everyone involved so much credit for all their hard work.

Having seen the play, I'm now very concerned about Cara being ready for the understudy performance on this Thursday, when she will be one of the leads. She will have lots of dialog and songs to perform. Most of the rehearsals have focused on the two girls who share this role for the six paid shows. Cara has been included in rehearsals, but has not actually had the same opportunity to practice this part. Now, she will have a few rehearsals after school before her performance this week. She has a great memory and I am sure she will handle the lines. However, the songs and choreography are going to be challenging and she is starting to become anxiety ridden.

The pre-show meltdown is coming. Though this theater work is what Cara wants to be involved in, I still cannot help worrying about how all this will go for her. You really have to have a strong love for performing to put yourself "out there" for everyone to watch. Jeepers, I couldn't do it! But I love that she can. By Sunday night we were all exhausted.

Monday was a "mixed bag." Vicki met me early for an indoor-mall walk. It was great to fit that exercise in again. After that I met my friend Colette for breakfast to celebrate her birthday. The reunion ended up with us coming back home to spend some extra time. We talked for hours; it was as though we hardly skipped a beat. Actually, we had not gotten together socially in almost twenty-three years. I am happy for her that she is happily remarried. Her daughter is certainly "the apple of her eye," and is attending a prestigious college.

It is funny when you know someone so well growing up; I still recall her family's dynamics. I am able to remember many childhood experiences that we shared together. Seeing Colette years later as a parent herself is interesting. I hope she was also feeling good about our time together today.

Vicki called me with some disturbing news. My mother and Irwin attended a meeting for Garry this morning. They were told that Garry's condition has become so serious, that he will have to be moved out of his group home and placed in a nursing home. Additionally, his workplace can no longer provide a job for him. He has lost functioning of his right hand and cannot write the messages down that he was able to take over the phone. He had been the official greeter and phone receptionist, and now people were having difficulty in understanding his speech. We understand how long they have put off this dismissal. Even so, it is heartbreaking news.

We are well aware how much more work his condition has placed on the people caring for him at home and work. Garry has always made such a great impression on everyone he comes in contact with, and they all regard him as a truly special human being. This is so painful for everyone.

Garry was devastated with this latest development. It is my mom's greatest fear to have him placed in a nursing home. We will try to concentrate on the fact that he will be where people are better prepared to handle and take care of him. It is vague as to how much time we have to find a new situation for him. My mom has had some year to deal with. As a mother myself, I cannot imagine how this is for her. This additional news is distressing and almost unbearable.

Later, I picked up Cara from her rehearsal—the "meltdown" had started. She is stressed to the max and yet, I know she will be fine. There was little I could do or say to help her. When we came home I made her a cup of tea, and insisted that she take a break before studying for her test tomorrow. I am a little worn out myself from this day.

This morning I met my Mom, Irwin and Vicki at the diner. It is my Mom's eighty-second birthday today, March 2nd. We did our best. Our concerns over Garry's health and the new developments regarding his living and job situations were getting to us all. Mom and Irwin went to visit my Aunt Betty after breakfast determined to enjoy the rest of the day as best they could. I ran around doing many of the things I successfully avoided this past weekend.

It was an afternoon of errands and cooking. When I picked Cara up from school she came out of the rehearsal looking much more comfortable and happier than she had the day before. It was a relief to hear that things had gone much better today. She has a field trip to go to tomorrow. Not being bogged down with homework tonight will be more relaxing for her.

This was day one of my shots for these four injections and I went to Loretta's house again. It did not hurt at all this time which was a nice surprise. However, about an hour or two into the evening I was already achy. The side effects of these shots are tough and I cannot wait until this is over and done with. It is evident that the injections keep the white cell count up. I feel strong and no doubt the shots are largely responsible.

My goals have been to keep to my chemo schedule and to go to the school play this year. Actually, the play has probably been a huge distraction and substantial motivation for me. When there are difficult things to deal with, and especially when they are as frustrating as with my brother's situation—it is important to make the most of the good times. *Sometimes we have to make a conscious effort not to diminish the other events that are going on.* It is still a blessing to share these times. I think it will be a tremendous boost for the rest of our family as well.

Since the school bus comes early, I have chosen to make extra trips to school in the morning to allow Cara to start the day a bit later. On the other end most days, I have to pick her up after practice. This schedule has kept me hopping. Counting down the weeks and days to the performances made me acutely aware how fast time does go by. Winter would have been so much longer for me without all this commotion. It was great to have the play to look forward to.

With the first successful weekend behind us now, we are looking ahead anxiously to Cara's big understudy lead performance. Vicki is going to try and come to this performance. She has never seen Cara in anything before. Vicki's germ phobia makes school a "bad place." It will be interesting watching her reaction to Cara's performance.

Keith is planning on missing one evening class and should be able to catch the train home for the show. That will mean a lot to Cara; we are looking forward to seeing him, too. Anne is definitely coming to this show. Cara does not know who is specifically coming because I did not want to freak her out completely. I will have a DVD of the regular show which will mean I can show Garry that one. It will not be Cara's understudy performance, but I know he will be eager to see it anyway. Today is the final rehearsal for the understudy show tomorrow night. I am getting nervous. Oy!!

Vicki and I walked this morning. We talked about Garry some more. It is so important that we can share these concerns together.

We both watched *Oprah* yesterday and we discussed the show's impact on us. Roger Ebert, the film critic of many years, was her guest. He has survived thyroid cancer. He is wheelchair-bound and cannot speak. He cannot eat foods as he is missing the lower jaw and the bottom of his mouth and he is nourished via IV. He has full use of his hands, so that he can continue to use his computer and type. This allows him to communicate and to continue to work. His magnificent spirit shone through his bright eyes and brilliant smile. His words which were audible through technology were so powerful and impressive. He said he felt, "Terrific!" and I believe that he does in his own unique way. He also said, "No more surgeries." They will not enable him to walk or eat. He is no longer concerned with changing his face through more surgical procedures.

To say he was inspirational is a gross understatement. He and his wife were amazing people. I was humbled by their love and strength. Wow!

When I picked up the girls at about 9:45 last night from their rehearsal it was unclear how things went from Cara's face. Her friend said, "Cara is an awesome actress." A little while after we returned home Cara seemed uncomfortable about one of the big numbers. She is lifted by a large group of boys who are dancing and running all over with her in the air. This is particularly tough for her as she has a fear of heights; being lifted off the ground takes her right out of her comfort zone. This number is long and lively. Cara is concerned she has not practiced it enough. Having seen the show I understand her apprehensions.

The big day is here. I drove Cara and a friend to school this morning. The girls were as focused on this morning's standardized test as they were on tonight's performance. Maybe they were not focused on either. Of course, I was focused enough for us all. The play's director is planning to work on the musical number that has been creating such angst after school for tonight's show. After this night, the remaining three performances will be much less stressful and I'm glad we are almost there.

After dropping the girls off, I met my sister at the mall to walk. Vicki and I mostly talked over Garry's situation. When that became too difficult we switched to thoughts of watching Cara later on.

Keith text messaged me that he is working on figuring out his schedule. He wants to see this particular show, but class times and train times may be very close at best. Keith has been involved with these high school productions from playing the drums in the pit orchestra throughout his high school years. Those were great experiences for him, and he understands that the understudy roles are a huge effort and compliment for the person who lands the opportunity.

I had been so focused on the understudy show that I forgot about today's shot. The nurse at the doctor's office suggested taking the injection out of the refrigerator to bring the medication to room temperature. This makes the injection hurt less or not at all. Loretta called to say she was home. I quickly took the injection and placed it on the table before I took Cara back to school for this evening's show. When I returned I went straight to Loretta. She asked me how I made out with last night's shot. Maybe it is that I am thinking about so many other things that I did not concentrate on how I was feeling today. We were both glad that apparently there were no problems and left it at that.

Keith came home by train. We picked him up at the station on our way to the high school. I was happy he made it. Keith felt confident in Cara's ability based on her last year's performance and he was psyched. Having not seen how nervous his sister was this week, made him calmer than John and I.

Grandma and Grandpa were already at the school as we expected. They are always early for these things. Anne and Dave were there, too. Soon Vicki joined us and I was jumping-out-of-my-skin nervous about the whole thing. We settled in our seats and the director came out first to announce that this was a rehearsal, and if necessary there might be interruptions to work on various parts.

Everything was great and better than we could have imagined. Cara was outstanding, and from her entrance on was delightful and very funny. The three understudies did so well that it seemed like the real deal. How Cara was able to get her part down with such few rehearsals was impressive. The number we were all concerned about came out great. A large group of boys, who are supposed to be with the Brazilian Navy, sing and dance to the Conga and pick Cara up and toss her around and around. It was absolutely screamingly funny! As with every performance there were little things that did not go as planned, but everything was fine. Cara seemed relieved and very pleased when it was over.

Grandma, Grandpa and Aunt Vicki had such a wonderful time. We were all thrilled we were able to share this experience together. We laughed so hard at times that tears were running down our faces. Everyone was excited the show was a success. Wow, we were all so proud of Cara. What a treat! She can cruise through the remaining three shows in her smaller roles and just enjoy them without the intense pressure of the last few days. Whew!

John, Keith, Cara and I came back home and sat around the kitchen table. Cara was still wound up and we had tea and talked. Anne came back after driving her boyfriend home and we all sat for a while longer. It was great as we have not all been together lately. Keith made himself his usual bowl of cereal. Then, he enjoyed some of the other goodies he has missed by not being at home. I'm a happy momma hen with all my chicks at home.

John had been concerned that this was a huge challenge Cara might not be ready for tonight. He had been abnormally nervous for her, but later he was relaxed and comfortable. All of us needed some all-out fun and this was more than we could have asked for. What a great night! It is comforting that no matter what else is going on you are able to fully enjoy these times. How sweet.

Keith needed to go back to school the next morning. There is one more week before his school break and he had to get going. We ate breakfast together and I asked him to go to the store with me to pick up several cases of water. It is a huge help for me when he does this. He left to go back to school shortly after that errand. Keith took his car and drove back this time. In a week he will have the convenience of bringing lots of laundry and other things home. It was a short visit this time, but it all worked out great.

Meanwhile Vicki met Mom, Irwin and Garry at the doctor's office this morning for a checkup. The doctor spoke to my brother about needing more care than he was receiving. It was another difficult meeting.

I took it easy today. Ginny called and I stopped over her house for a cup of tea and a quick visit with her. We both said the slightly improved weather made us feel encouraged that we would soon be able to walk outside again.

Later I went to Loretta's for my last shot of this week. Yay, only one more round of these!

Unfortunately, I feel like I have been exposed to so many people with colds this past week. When someone tells me how sick they are while they are in my face it makes me crazy. Obviously, they are pretty sure that I will notice it anyway. Keith also had a mild sore throat. Lots of the time it is more allergies related with him. I cannot be sure which it is now. Loretta's husband was sick and he made himself scarce when I went over for my shot. I have been in their home for a brief time each day for the last four days.

It has been a terrible week for getting sleep. Between the show craziness and my concerns about my brother, I am tired and not sleeping well. I feel a little edgy and I am thinking maybe I pushed my luck. I am having serious mouth side effects this time. The roof of my mouth is swollen and sore and my tongue is the same. The special mouth wash medicine is not as effective yet. There are a moderate amount of general aches, although it is not as bad as it has been at other times. I am tired and moody from several days of all this and the extra running around.

Although I skipped Friday night's performance, I saw the last two performances on Saturday. Mom and Irwin had tickets for the matinee show and I decided see that one at the last minute. John quickly showed me how to use the video camera and I thought it would be a perfect opportunity to get some of the show on film. It was especially important because I wanted to show Garry something from the show as soon as possible.

The night performance was the lead cast that had not performed since last weekend. A couple of our supportive neighbors attended this performance. The audience was great and every actor ended the weekend with a terrific and very special effort. Cara had her smallest part and even so it was all tremendous fun! We are so happy for everyone involved with the show.

John and I had a rare weekend breakfast out. It was just us and we felt like things had gone so well that a little celebration was in order. Later we were all exhausted. I tried to watch the Academy Awards show I usually love. After our school's theater success of the past two weekends, this Oscar-business was not so exciting to me. Certainly after the craziness of this past year, it just did not matter as much.

THE GOOD AND THE BAD

Vicki and I met at the park. It was a gorgeous, chilly morning, but temperatures were headed toward sixty-degrees. We started our walk even earlier this morning as Vicki had business appointments for the day. I went with several layers of clothing. It was lovely to be walking outside again.

We were anxious to find out how Garry made out on a test today. They are trying to determine why he is choking and coughing so much. It is called a "swallow test." The group home and office staff are concerned that they cannot continue to take care of him adequately. We know the answer to that question. However, we are concerned about his emotional well-being, and know what these changes will mean to his sense of security.

Things went poorly because Garry could not complete the test; they are thinking that he may need a feeding tube. Oh my God, this just keeps getting worse! Another meeting is scheduled for today, and I feel terrible that Mom and Irwin will be there without Vicki and me. I am scheduled to see my doctor about the same time.

The social worker called Vicki and told her that the recommendation was made to change Garry's living situation. They are looking for a facility to take him as soon as possible. Understanding this problem does not make it any easier on anyone. The social worker told my sister, "If you find another place he can be moved again." This arrangement could be a temporary quick fix. Truthfully, I don't believe anything can be done easily once this move is made and I am scared for him.

It is impossible to think of Garry in these circumstances. Mom and I talked which is not very easy lately. She was venting and asked, "Why is this happening to him?" and I told her, "I never ask *why* because no answer would be sufficient, or acceptable. Instead I am choosing to be thankful that he led his life as he has until now. He made the most of what he was given; he has actually been more successful than most of us. Garry has been a wonderful person who everyone adores." She agreed but remains frightened for him and I understood.

Anne came home for a rare dinner with John and me. I told her about the newest developments. She had been planning to stop by Garry's for a while and just had not managed yet. Immediately she decided to go over to see him, and brought the video camera to show him some of Cara's performance from last week. We called him ahead and he was thrilled to expect the visit.

Later Anne called me, obviously upset about her uncle's general health. Although warned, she was still shocked at the further deterioration of his condition. Her friend, who was fond of Garry, met her for the visit. It was thoughtful and I was quite impressed by the gesture. He brought my brother a bottle of Coke, as it is Garry's favorite. They had a nice time together. After Anne left my brother called me right away to say how good it was to see them.

Garry mentioned that Anne showed him a picture of her new boyfriend. In true form he said, "I did not say anything to her, but you know how I feel about the long-hair thing." He would have all males carefully buzzed every two or three weeks. As weak as he sounded, he is still Garry. I spoke to my mom later and she is starting to accept that changes are necessary.

Everyone, including my brother, is reminding me that tomorrow will be a huge day for me. It is my last chemotherapy. However, my thoughts are much more with the events surrounding Garry tomorrow.

My appointment for this last treatment was in the afternoon on March 10, 2010. Vicki and I arrived in the city earlier than necessary, which allowed us plenty of time to get my bloodwork out of the way. Then we went to have a little lunch before my appointment. We had just placed our order when I was surprised by my niece Jennifer, who was there to help celebrate my last chemo day. I had not seen her in quite a while and this was a nice surprise. It was sweet of her to take the time today.

We had a delicious lunch. No pizza today and we had a good visit together. Afterward Jen walked with us to get Vicki her tea. She left us to make one stop at the Museum of Modern Art to see an exhibit she had wanted to catch. Lunch was the perfect acknowledgement of the importance of this day.

As expected, the schedule at the doctor's office was fairly busy. The staff was quite aware that this was my last treatment. Each person I spoke with congratulated me and asked if there was any celebration planned. I told them we had met my niece for lunch; and that I was very happy this was the last treatment. There is still one more round of injections in about ten days from now. My agenda today did not include thinking of running out for a celebration just yet. All I kept thinking was, *This is a big day in my journey!* It is a relief to know chemo is completed and that it went smoothly.

My doctor was pleased with my bloodwork results and offered me a hug and congratulations. She was glad to hear that I scheduled my operation for early May. She remarked about the fact that I had been a great patient. On my next appointment in one month we will consult on my future course of action, and she will order more detailed bloodwork.

I told her she could give my name and phone number to any patient who needs to speak to someone who has recently gone through this standard treatment. The doctor thanked me and explained, "Other patients have made the same offer and rarely does anyone take advantage of it." As I reflect on that, I guess I would rather not have that responsibility really.

We waited a while before the chemo suite was ready and then we were called in. The nurse used the vein in my arm, which has been a problem at times. Shortly after inserting the needle I had to complain about the intensifying pain. Next we used the vein from my hand, which has been more successful recently. Vicki and I watched *Oprah* and before we knew it treatment number eight was over. Thank Goodness this is all behind me now!

When I got home everyone else in my family seemed quite relieved that the treatments were completed. There was almost a collective sigh of relief. That evening I was careful to drink my fluids and as usual the day left me worn out. The next morning I noticed the same slight strange stomach, and a bit of that "off" feeling that I experienced last time. I forgot to ask the doctor if this might have been the different anti-nausea drug prior to the chemo drugs. It may just be the accumulative effect of the chemo treatments.

Despite how I felt, Vicki and I met for an early walk. Then, I had an appointment to get my hair cut mid-morning. After that, I felt energetic and stopped by Ginny's for a visit, which was good. There was one more quick errand and I went back home to take it easy. I decided the food store would have to wait for another day, as I just ran out of steam.

Truthfully, I think that my anxiety about Garry has taken more out of me than anything else has. He is going to the Wound Center to have a bed sore checked out today. There seems to be some particular concern regarding this situation by the staff at Garry's home. Anne had noticed her uncle's discomfort the other night when she visited there.

My mother seems convinced that the process of getting him into a nursing home will still take some time. The social worker said that they will help with finding a facility.

Garry's checkup went better than expected. They medicated and cleaned the area which the center did not think was that serious. They suggested a special cushion to sit on which may be helpful. We are all pleased for Garry that there was no emergency today. We'll see how the next few days shape up.

Last night was more uncomfortable than usual for me. My stomach was not right and I thought constipation was likely the problem. However, by the time I went to bed I noticed that my cheeks were ruddy-looking. I woke up feeling slightly better. There are a few errands that I need to take care of today, but afterward it will be a quiet day. It is a dreary, rainy day and that seems like a fairly good plan.

WEATHER AND OTHER STORMS

There is so much to catch up on in my journal. It has actually been about two weeks since I made an entry. In that time we experienced a tremendous storm. The first Saturday brought severe wind and rain, and by about seven in the evening we lost our electricity. My mom called on her cell phone earlier to report the same situation at her house.

Cara was across town with a group of friends from the afternoon on, and called to say she could stay overnight with the group. As we had no electricity, and they had *not* lost their power that seemed reasonable. The weather was ferocious and we were relieved not to go out to pick her up. When we looked out our window we could see lights in the sky from exploding transformers. It was weird and then, we heard the sounds of sirens all around us.

My sister, Paul and Jen were crazy enough to venture out early in the evening to grab a bite to eat. Vicki called from the road to report that there were trees down and power outages in much of the area. When she returned home she found no power and a tree had fallen on her home causing a substantial amount of exterior damage. What a mess!

Never do I recall anything as extensive as this happening before. Thank goodness we all had cell phones. It was a challenge recharging our phones outside our home; having these phones to get through the next few days was a tremendous comfort.

We used candles, flashlights, and lots of extra clothing to manage through the next three days. During days one and two, we were very careful to keep the refrigerator door closed as much as possible. We were luckier than some people in that we had hot water and we could use our stove because they are both powered by gas. Even so, when the house temperature is about fifty degrees, it gets pretty nasty. The most comfortable place was under the covers.

This made us realize how horrific the conditions of the disasters that we have heard about must really be. Even with a roof over our heads, food, water and more, we were terribly uncomfortable. It is unimaginable how the victims of New Orleans, the tsunami and Haiti's earthquake made it through. I am embarrassed even to say how difficult our inconveniences felt to us.

By day three, we were staying out of the house as much as we could. It definitely thrilled me to take six loads of laundry to a warm laundromat and spend a couple of hours there. Keith came home Sunday morning after spending a night at school with no power and was on a school break for the week. That was a help because John had been working desperately to keep our sump-pump working. Our backup battery system was not working well and required constant attention. He ended up ripping the battery out of his car in the middle of the heaviest time of the rain and wind, and replaced the one in the pump that went dead.

The next morning the weather was barely improved, and many trees closed off roads. Flooding made traveling quite difficult. John had to go out in my car and buy another battery to replace the old one. Then, he put his car battery back in his car. He ran back and forth to his brother's home to recharge the batteries as frequently as he could. As he says, "It was a fire drill." It all worked out in the end and we realized how fortunate we were.

Our power was out for almost seventy-two hours. Five bags of food from two refrigerators and freezers had to be thrown into the garbage. Some of that should have been gone before this event. I am particularly careful now as chemotherapy leaves your stomach more sensitive. The body is depleted of some of the good stuff needed to fight off problems that you might normally be able to handle. When our power returned we were all thrilled!

My mom went to her sister Betty's condo one night. The next night, we had power and Mom and Irwin were planning to stay with us. This plan sent me into a panic! I immediately went into major clean-up mode. After several hours we were set to have guests camp-out for whatever time was needed. As it turned out, they made a stop to their home and found power restored. Their house was cold, and the land-line phone still out; while it warmed up they came to us for only a couple of hours. We lucked out because we were prepared to help and then it wasn't necessary. Hey, we ended up with a cleaner house.

Vicki and Paul and their dog spent several nights at a local motel before their power was restored. Jen had gone back to Manhattan on the Sunday of the storm. Anne also chose not to be in a home with no power, and she stayed with a friend. Vicki's power returned after five days. Besides the tree damage, the compressor on her refrigerator broke down. She was stressed from the whole situation; yet, she was able to put it all in perspective. My sister kept going which is certainly her MO.

Mary and Bob, who live ten minutes away, had only lost power a few hours; we ended up storing my injections in their refrigerator. If we had been more realistic we would have brought lots of our food there early on. I assumed that power would be restored much sooner. After a while, you are not sure if it is too long a time to save much of what you have anyway.

John's Aunt Betty about twenty-minutes away was fine and with power. Thank goodness Garry's home also had no problems; we were all relieved about that. The rest of the week and some time beyond, the entire area was slowly being cleaned up and repaired. It was bizarre.

After dealing with all of the weather-related messes, we then had to get back to the most serious issue that faced our family, which was my brother. Everyone was exhausted and overwhelmed. I made it through all my chemo appointments, and I was ready to insert myself into the task of finding an acceptable nursing home.

My mom seemed to be waiting for assistance from Garry's group home social worker and manager. It was all confusing as to what and when things needed to be done. She found the whole business intolerable, and was probably trying to convince herself that this situation was not imminent. Occasionally a conversation ended with her saying, "Do you know how hard this is for me? I can't talk about this anymore!"

Finally, I had a complete blowup. When my mother declared, "I would rather die than see this happen to Garry," I flipped out! Hopefully, I will never have to face anything like this with one of my own children. Although I understood, I felt this defense was going to make it nearly impossible for us to be more productive.

My greatest fear is that there will be an emergency situation where Garry gets thrown into a home only because they have an "opening." Ideally we should place applications only where we are most comfortable in regard to his care. Garry's speech is getting much more difficult to understand. The thought of Mom and Irwin, at ages eighty-two and eighty-eight, driving long distances frequently is an additional concern. A fairly convenient location where we can keep a close eye on him would be preferable.

I believe it is critical to place my brother soon. This will allow the caregivers to get to know what a special person he is. I am convinced that

Garry will charm his way into their lives. Right now, he is still able to tell us what is going on when we are not with him.

Anyway, Mom and I blew off some steam and with Irwin's help we worked it out. Our hard feelings were mended quickly and we got right on track again. We have even managed to spend a week running around to various nursing homes together and found two acceptable facilities. It is still horrible to think of Garry in these places; he would be the youngest resident by far in either home. We agree that he needs better and more appropriate attention now and for the rest of his life. It is just a matter of timing and luck now. We hope that one of these two homes will take him.

Legal matters were also needed to be taken care of this week; we spoke to Mom and Irwin's lawyer and he reviewed things for us. We needed to draw up a Medical Advanced Directive. A friend helped us out as she is a notary. She was happy to come with me to my brother's home and have him sign papers in front of her there; this was a great help. Garry had a couple of doctors' visits already this week and he did not need more treks out.

My friend was so touched by how friendly and sharp Garry was despite everything else that he was dealing with. She remarked in the car on the way back home, "Remind me about what's up with Garry? He is so with-it mentally speaking." It is clear that eventually he will be trapped in his body. My friend understood my feelings, and she recognized the extraordinary and special person my brother is.

I talked Garry into allowing me to take his two bulletin boards and his entire standing, framed photos collection home with me. I promised him that I would quickly return all of them newly arranged in large poster frames. He was compliant, though I think he thought it unnecessary. Last Sunday, I noticed these things were way out of control and that he couldn't see most of the pictures from his chair. The dresser he sits facing as he watches TV was topped with lots of dusty frames.

I maniacally cut and pasted these pictures. Other older family photos were added which I thought he would enjoy looking at. All the pictures were put in two large poster frames. One of the posters was all family, plus a few very close friends, who are like family. The other poster was all pictures of his friends. The next day, I returned the new posters and placed them standing on the top of his dresser where he could clearly see them. He was thrilled with the newly arranged pieces. It made me feel so good that he was delighted with the results. These are "new" in one sense, but by the time he needs to relocate they will be familiar to him. They will be a perfect touch to help personalize his new accommodations.

It is anticipated that all of the good memories and pictures of people that he cares for and loves will bring him comfort in days to come. My brother thoroughly enjoys showing off family and friends photos. This worked out great. The bulletin boards also went back up where they had hung before with small posters re-hung on them. The room looked much better except that the large framed pieces now covered the mirror over the dresser. Garry was even more pleased as he said, "I wanted to take the mirrors away because I don't like to look at myself anyway."

The group home's manager needed to have my brother sign an application. This man had been very helpful and we knew he would continue to be of assistance as changes occurred. I agreed to make his job easier and I asked my brother to sign the papers. It caused Garry to voice some concerns and we spoke a while together. He recalled news stories on the subject of nursing homes and said, "You *always* hear bad things about those places." I tried to reassure him that we were being careful; we would only apply to ones we felt comfortable about. It was obvious that he was frightened.

My brother and I talked about how the move would provide improved care and more activities for him when he can no longer work. Of course, he feels his present care is fine and would prefer to stay where he is. Garry said, "I don't want to stop working." He appeared more visibly upset about when his work might end. He does understand that the choice is not ultimately his or ours; he knows that the decision has already been made to find a nursing home. I left feeling his appreciation for my efforts. My guess is that he desperately needed to talk about these things. He wasn't fighting the plan; he simply had concerns to voice.

The group home was getting ready for a birthday party that night for one of the residents. I left feeling everything was OK for now.

Later that evening at about 10:00 Garry called me. I was sure he was going to thank me again as is his style. Instead he told me that his girlfriend had been over for the party and that she told him, "I don't want a boyfriend who cannot walk anymore." He was shocked at her remark and then commented to me, "Who would have known that she was a hardhearted bitch!" My brother almost never uses a curse word, but he was very hurt. I was stunned and upset for him. I know the remark came from a mentally challenged individual; yet, I could not imagine anyone being so insensitive and callous.

Garry then told me that he called another former ex-girlfriend and they are back together. Wow, now what could I say? I laughed at how quickly he rebounded. Then, I teased him, "I don't know Garr—you may be a little fickle in the romance department?" Then he asked to speak to Cara and went into this whole thing with her. She basically was left similarly open-jawed. Vicki had shut her phone off to recharge it and was not able to be reached. Mom was out as she and Irwin had purchased tickets long ago for a show. They were unavailable to receive this news. My mom might have gone ballistic at hearing the poorly chosen comment. Maybe not to Garry, but some lucky person would have gotten an earful.

This morning when I spoke with my mother I told her about Garry and his girlfriend. She was not unhappy. I did not give the details as I did not want to hear her comments. Garry most likely will tell Mom, so she can say the things that he is thinking and would rather not say. On one hand, I totally forgive this person for not knowing better; still, I am saddened that my brother had to endure her comments. Jeepers, this is so unfair!

—⁂—

I was able to speak with Laura this week. Her husband is going to need some surgery soon and I am concerned about them. She promised to keep me informed, and we are still going to try to get together soon.

My high school friend Carol sent me a little note which always makes the day feel a bit brighter. Colette called on Tuesday and we decided that she will probably see my brother after Easter. I saw Ginny a couple of times during the past week. She had a huge family party last weekend and now, seemed to be coming down with a cold. The weather has been a mixed-bag and I haven't managed to walk with any of my pals.

Yay! March 23 started my last round of injections. Loretta is really busy, and so we have done the shots at all different times of the day. They are easier than usual, and I am hoping the medication survived our power loss last week. John read the information that comes inside the box of injections, and he was sure they were fine at the temperature that the refrigerator thermometer displayed. I told Loretta that John and I want to take them out to dinner to celebrate the end of my chemo and to thank her. I will never forget her generous assistance. I will go over to her in just a few minutes for the last shot. *Excuse me while I do a little dance!*

When I came home from Loretta's, Mom called and asked if they could come over to use our land-line phone. Their phone repair was not done again today. When they came I could see how frustrated they both were, and I suggested that I give the complaint department a try. To my surprise Irwin eagerly agreed to this plan. After a half-hour of mostly waiting on hold I finally connected with supervisor. I explained my parents' particular circumstances. I was insistent that this repair be made quickly. I reminded the phone company representative that the service was already out for weeks. She said, "The repair was on the schedule for today and it could be resolved in the next two hours."

Mom and Irwin left feeling we had done everything possible for today. John and I left for a school fundraiser. I could have skipped this, but I thought this forced break was wise.

The rest of the weekend was quiet. Saturday morning, I had to call the phone company again to report that the repair had not been done the day before. This time I was directed to a supervisor. The conversation was calmer. The person who spoke with me was very reasonable and we talked for quite a while. She explained all the damage that still needed to be taken care of before certain repairs could be completed. She told me of the large number of customers that were in the same circumstances, and explained that they were all emergencies at this point. It all made sense. I explained the difficulty my parents were already overwhelmed by and added that they were also "cell-phone challenged." She understood, as her elderly mother was the same way.

The supervisor promised that she would reschedule the repair and "stay on top of it" personally. She called back a little while later with a time to expect the repairman. Before long, I was pleased to hear from my mom that repairmen were on the job. Halleluiah, the phone finally was fixed! Mom and Irwin were so relieved. They fully credited me for the success. Maybe it happened because of my persistence, or maybe it would have happened anyway. A "thank you" to that supervisor is probably more in order.

Monday morning Vicki and I were thrilled to meet for an early walk. The heavy rains were with us for a couple of days more. As the weather became uglier, I was happy to be in for the rest of the day.

Keith called to let us know he will be home on Sunday for the week break from school. He has a rugby game on Saturday which he seems very excited about. He says his shoulder is good, but I will still worry about him playing this exceptionally rough game.

It is the first night of Passover and I am feeling guilty that I am not planning to do anything for the holiday this year. Truthfully, I am not up to handling the task. It is definitely an emotional decision more than a physical one. This is a tough year and without Garry's attendance the celebration is especially difficult. Although I always say that I am non-practicing, I often make this dinner. It is my way of remembering the enjoyment my Dad always had on this particular holiday. He loved to abbreviate the event down to a simple, but traditional meal with just enough readings from the prayer book to make it official and meaningful. Irwin and Mom enjoy keeping to this particular holiday, too.

John's brother Tom and his wife Barbara were hosting Easter. Mary and Bob will be there, as well as some of my sister-in-law Barbara's family. Mom and Irwin will spend that day with Vicki, Paul and Jennifer. I think this will work well for everyone.

It was nice not to be knee-deep in preparations. We contributed various goodies. The day was made more enjoyable as Tom and Barb's youngest grandchild was there. Babies bring such joy. Although, it also reminded me about what an exhausting time that is. Everything was great. We all pitched in to help out. Barbara's sister and her family were there as well. The different people created a new mix for this Easter day. Keith ended up catching the train back to school around 8:30. That enabled him to spend the entire day with us. I was glad not to make the holiday trip back on the highway, which was jammed with traffic.

Mom and Irwin visited my brother early Easter afternoon. Later they met Vicki, Paul and Jen for dinner at a local restaurant. We made the best of this holiday week, which felt stressful for everyone. We knew Garry wanted to be with us. We all agreed not to take the risk of bringing him out as he was not up to that anymore. This saddened everyone.

It was going to be a hectic week or more ahead. My appointment with the oncologist is on Wednesday. Then, I will see the plastic surgeon on Thursday. Following those visits will be the gynecologist's appointment on Monday. This was to set everything up for my next surgery in one month. I am becoming nervous about the double procedure.

MOVING ALONG

This was going to be a demanding week with Cara off from school. In addition to my doctors' appointments, Cara had a scheduled annual physical. Also I still wanted to visit Garry. Cara and I went by to see him Monday afternoon for a little while. He was excited to see his niece.

We brought him a strawberry milk shake and he completely enjoyed the drink despite the elimination of the real fruit. It still caused him to choke, which made us uncomfortable. Coincidentally, Mom and Irwin came by for a visit while we were there. The day was beautiful and we stayed outside with the other residents of the group home. It was great to see my brother out of his room. This seemed to perk him up a bit in general. While we were visiting a couple of women, who live across the street, came over to say "hello." The younger was the daughter who was caring for her ninety-four year old mother. They were friendly. They told us they have often talked with my brother through the years and they were concerned about him.

The daughter told us a little about the neighborhood, as they had lived there for a long time. She also included stories about her mother's experiences working in an amusement park when she was a young woman. Apparently her mother was the magician's assistant. Who would have guessed! The daughter described her mom's work. Her mother was the assistant who was sawed in half, and had been levitated; she was also responsible for other unusual jobs. Well, I guess they knew how to get our attention alright. Oh, my! If I were older this may have been the job for me. Their stories certainly made our visit interesting.

I am glad we got over to see Garry while Cara was off this week from school. He is weak and is speaking at a much lower volume. Even so my brother is still telling jokes. When you ask him, "What's new?" his answer is always, "New York, New Jersey . . ." He asked us how Easter was and said, "It must have been hare-raising." He loves those kinds of puns. He is amazing!

Vicki and I walked Monday and Tuesday. We knew the rest of the week might be more difficult. Wednesday, April 7, we went in to see the oncologist. This was a post-chemo visit. There was the normal routine exam, and a brief discussion with my doctor. She ordered bloodwork completed to evaluate how I am now that chemo is finished. She wants me to come back to see her after my surgery next month. Then, I start on the five-year drug which will block any estrogen from stimulating the production of any breast cancer cells. Although I remembered speaking with her regarding this plan months ago, I am leery of medications used over long periods.

Gee whiz, a double mastectomy, chemotherapy, an oophorectomy and now a five-year pill regime, this is too much! We are still talking about *this* breast cancer. It feels like it never ends.

Vicki had an uncharacteristically bad day. She was hit with several serious business problems all at once, and was trying to handle them by phone and take care of my appointment. She is always able to work around these things very adeptly; however, this was not easily managed today. It made me feel terribly guilty. Unfortunately, there are more appointments coming up this next week and probably for a couple of months. To top this excursion off, when we picked up our car at the lot Vicki's foot was hit by someone's heavy luggage which fell over on her. She believes that she attracted this negative event. I believed it was a bad day. As always, all worked out and there were only survivors.

That same day was Anne's 25th birthday, April 7. We talked and I told Anne that I would have Grandma and Grandpa and Vicki and Paul over next weekend to celebrate. Since I had my appointment, which had taken away a chunk of the day, and Mom and Irwin had a meeting concerning my brother, this seemed reasonable. After a birthday dinner out with several friends, Anne brought them back home to watch a TV program they are all hooked on.

This allowed me the rare opportunity to try my hand at baking a cake for the occasion. It is so unlike me to do this. In my family I am known as "the Bakery Maven." Anne was so pleased that I made her a cake. It was well worth the work to see her appreciation. It was fun and I must admit it came out pretty well. Anne liked the clothes I picked out, too. I felt like a winner. It was also nice to see her friends again. Wow, it is wild to see them all grown up. It's all good.

Uncle Garry made his birthday call to Anne wishing her well and sending his love as always. He never forgets an occasion, and usually calls everyone else in the family to remind them to do the same. Truth be told, he is better at that sort of thing than most of us are. He even remembers our friends' birthdays and reminds us of those as well.

DETAILS, DISTRACTIONS AND DISTURBANCES

Today's appointment, April 8, was with my plastic surgeon. Vicki's day of dilemmas seemed to have worked out and she was in a "better place" today.

We expected that this appointment would be short and sweet. This particular doctor is never one to make any extra conversation and is usually on schedule. First, a woman came in and spoke to us explaining all the details of the operation that we needed to know about. That could have gone better, but we started off on the wrong foot with each other. I have to say that generally speaking, I am a very good patient. This woman abruptly began rattling off information about the procedures and details regarding this next operation. She spoke with the authority of a doctor and I was confused by this.

About two or three minutes into her speech I insisted on knowing who she was. Instead of an introduction, or an apology she looked at me almost shocked and asked, "You don't remember me? I am sure we must have met already." We had not. She announced that she was my doctor's head-nurse, and quickly stated she must have been away at the time of the earlier surgery. After that, things went downhill. She mentioned that the operation would take approximately one hour on each side. That fact surprised me as I thought this was going to be a very simple procedure. Apparently, there is a bit of tissue from the healing and scarring which is cut away before the implant exchange is completed. There will be sutures placed to create a fold under the implants making a more natural appearance under my breasts. The doctor will leave one drain on each side, which will not be placed as deeply as in the first operation.

The nurse also suggested an allergy specialist should check to make sure that I was really allergic to penicillin. This extra step just pushed the wrong button with me. It struck that raw nerve that does not want any more additional doctor's appointments or procedures. I kicked up a fuss at the suggestion. Actually, when I thought about this later it was not a bad idea. No one has ever suggested this before and that bothered me, too. I may have experienced a problem with the substitute antibiotic after my mastectomy and it was not a bad idea. I just wished this had been suggested earlier.

The plastic surgeon's nurse imparted various instructions for before and after the next surgery. She also remarked, "The gynecologist will be the one to decide if an overnight stay is appropriate after the oophorectomy." Maybe that doctor will be able to tell me more on Monday's appointment. Obviously, I am starting to freak out about this whole deal!

We spoke with other trained personnel in the doctor's office today whose credentials escape me now, and they filled us with facts and post surgery instructions. What surprised me most was that these implants won't necessarily last the rest of my life. Wow, I must be nuts because that never occurred to me. I recall hearing that MRI testing was necessary in fairly regular intervals through the years, to check the condition of the implants. But, more operations for replacements never entered my mind as anything but a rarity. If the implant was damaged in some way of course, replacement would be needed. Well was there a better choice for me? I guess not. Though there have been moments when I wondered if I could have done without them . . . that option was actually given almost no thought.

Cara and I went to her annual physical checkup. We talked with her doctor a little while about my situation and how it affects her. The doctor was not afraid of the subject; at the same time it was important information but nothing to dwell on now.

We all tried to will the height measurement one more inch taller, but in the end Cara was still barely four feet and eleven inches. The doctor emphasized, "Good things come in small packages." Yeah, that is not as comforting as you might think. Afterward, we did some errands together until a friend called Cara and invited her over. Spring break is over!

Just when I thought I had enough to think about this week, a call came from my oncologist's nurse late this afternoon. She informed me that my blood work showed a rise in my bilirubin count, which has something to do with red blood cells and the liver.

Boy, I'm having more and more fun and worries. I spoke with Vicki who reminded me that after the chemo and injections maybe, it is not so surprising or unusual to see some changes in the blood. She suggested that I try not to jump to any conclusions. This information was shared quickly with her as my schedule also affects her.

I desperately need a break from all this medical stuff. It is one of the few moments I feel like crying. It is not because I am feeling sorry for myself. Geez, I am getting scared—I don't like this!

John and I, and Loretta and her husband went out for dinner on Saturday night to thank her for helping me with all my injections. They are such nice people and very easy company. They chose to introduce us to a restaurant that we were unfamiliar with. I was glad to have an opportunity to show my appreciation, though this gesture was certainly inadequate.

Sunday evening we had Mom, Irwin, Vicki, Paul, Anne and Dave over to celebrate Anne's birthday. Keith was not able to come home; and Cara had a school trip into the city to see another play. We decided to BBQ. We had the meal and some more birthday cake. It was a good end to Anne's birthday.

Vicki and I headed into the city for my gynecological appointment on Monday, April 12. First, I went to the blood lab to repeat the blood test. Then we went for my scheduled appointment. As with the plastic surgeon, the gynecologist originally seemed casual about this surgery scheduled after the other procedure the same day, but not so much so today. This made me a bit uncomfortable as I initially got the impression that it *was* done fairly often. I know the idea of one-surgery day, as opposed to two-days, appealed to me, but I did not concoct the plan. Now, thinking of the dual recovery, I am wondering about this a little more. Hmmm?

Anyway, this surgeon said his part should take approximately forty-five minutes. The only thing will be how he will take the ovaries and tubes out. He does not know if he can do a laparoscopic procedure. My abdominal scar tissue from a previous surgery might create problems. If this is not possible he will make approximately two to three small incisions. He will also make sure there are no issues with my uterus requiring more surgery, which is fairly unlikely.

The doctor's fellow-assistant explained the surgery and what I need to do before and after that procedure. The doctor did make it clear to me that my ovaries produce very little estrogen now. However, estrogen is still produced in the glands. The five-year pill blocks estrogen, which can stimulate more breast cancer cells. He restated, "You have a thirty percent increased chance of having ovarian cancer by age seventy because of the BRCA 2 gene." He was very confident that the benefits of doing this procedure far outweigh the risks. OK, then "it's on."

Vicki and I were both stressed out and we went straight back to New Jersey. She was almost late for an appointment. Things are getting too wild and I am looking forward to getting this all behind me.

One nice thing about this week was that I got to spend some time with Ginny. We met for a couple of walks, which I desperately needed. Vicki is having cold or allergy problems plus a work week that is crazy. We haven't been able to get out and exercise together. It is important for me that for the next few weeks I stay as strong and healthy as possible. The doctor's nurse called to tell me my bloodwork came back with a good count and no problems. That was excellent news.

Colette called and we decided that we would meet next Friday and go to visit my brother together. I probably will not tell him until that day as to not risk disappointing him should the plan change. It is something that will surprise and please him. He has known Colette his whole life.

I visited Garry this afternoon. He seemed a little more comfortable, stronger and in better spirits then he has for a while now. It was so great to see this improvement in him. Mom, Irwin and Irwin's son Alan came by for a short visit while I was there. Alan came in from Colorado as he is concerned about Mom and his dad. It was nice that he saw Garry while he was feeling a little better than usual.

Garry was happy to see them, but suspicious that they were going to have dinner nearby at his favorite Jewish deli. Mom tried to deny it; however that was not believable to any of us.

Today, I met my friend Laura at a hospital nearby where she was waiting for news of her husband's surgery. He was having a biopsy to confirm a diagnosis he had gotten recently.

Laura was not sure whether she really needed or wanted any company. I convinced her that I could simply wait while her husband was in surgery and not intrude in any way. I know that I do not want to see more than one or two people in particular during these experiences. I wanted to be respectful of his needs; and I wanted to "be there" for my friend. After a quick stop to bring us some lunch, I met Laura. We waited for the doctor to talk with her after the procedure.

The doctor finally stepped in the waiting area and Laura got up to meet him. He walked her around the corner to talk more privately with her. They spoke for five minutes or so before she returned. I knew from her expression that it was serious news; it was not what they expected at all. The doctor told her that Artie has lymphoma, which seemed to be much more disturbing information.

My heart sank as I thought about their crisis; I remained calm and supportive. Laura was very concerned about how Art would handle this news; and I could feel her mind racing through different scenarios. Damn, this life gets more and more difficult! Of course, they are already added to my many prayers.

After the hospital I went home and I felt deeply upset about my friends. It did not occur to me that I was becoming more anxious and angry as the day went on. Later, I had to take care of errands before the start of the weekend. While at the gas station I got into an argument with the attendant. He has been there a couple of years, and when I see this fellow I try to avoid stopping there.

Today, this incompetent person had taken me "over the edge." When the boss came to see what had happened I was still angry. I told him emphatically, "This man is terrible at his job and I am in no mood for this today." Surely, I looked more unreasonable than anything else. I admit I handled the situation poorly. I was frustrated as it had been a long time in coming. Many times I have wanted to complain about this fellow, and yet I was sensitive that it might cost him his job. Oh well, guess I will be buying my gas elsewhere from now on.

Now, I realize how disturbed I am becoming regarding all the problems that are popping up around me. I have to be more careful before more things get out of control. This was a bad day. *A really, awful day!*

Monday, April 19, Colette and I went to see Garry and after all my efforts to surprise him, I actually goofed that up a bit. He was sitting out in front of his house as we approached him from behind. His manager announced my walking toward him with a friend. Instantly, I made the introductions between Colette and the manager. Despite my original intentions, Garry heard of Colette's presence before he actually saw her. In any case he was tickled to see her.

Colette had been nervous about seeing her old friend's condition in person, and worried that she might become visibly distressed. Garry quickly used all his tricks and showed his delight for the visit. This brought her great relief and eased her apprehensions. They sat chatting away about her family and he frequently noted how beautiful Colette is. He covered all the important bases before the visit ended. His remarks included her mom and her daughter's beauty too. My brother didn't miss a trick!

Garry's many clear memories of childhood details were impressive. He also reminded Colette that she once owned an old green Mustang, which she seemed to remember fondly. It was a good visit, and we were all grateful that we were able to enjoy the time together.

Mom and Irwin stopped by in the middle of our visit and they were equally glad to catch up with their former neighbor. I know my mom appreciated this effort very much. It made us all feel that special bond, which comes from years and years of knowing each other. We all felt a little better. We might be able to get together once more before surgery, but I am not sure.

SIDETRACKED

The plan for next week is about everything that I want to take care of before my surgery. There are the much-needed cleaning jobs that should be addressed before surgery. After all, it might be some time before I would be physically up to certain tasks. Now, my standards are not as high as they should be and these things were not entirely attracting my efforts. No matter what else had to be done this week, I should include some more walking as it will keep me healthier through surgery.

Thank goodness it is the weekend. I am not going to tackle much of any of these things the next couple of days. Yes, I am a great procrastinator!

The weekend was fairly busy between Yankees' baseball and socializing a bit. We met Mom, Irwin, Alan, Vicki and Paul for dinner on Saturday at a local Italian restaurant. We caught up on all Alan's family-news, and spent a pleasant and calm couple of hours.

Sunday we decided to have Greg and Ginny over for dinner. It is always wonderful to spend time with them so that was a pleasure. Just as they were due to arrive John's boyhood buddy Lou stopped by. We invited him to stay and he joined us for dinner also. We had not seen him in a while as he moved out of the area last year. He had come this way for a funeral wake visit today. We had a relaxing BBQ and a good time. It was April 25 and only twelve more days until my surgery and I'm thankful for this weekend's burst of social events.

The to-do list was being carefully constructed and defined. It was becoming clearer that I was overwhelmed by the tasks, the fleeting time and life's various stresses.

Before long I was allowing myself to be sidetracked again. These were of the shopping kind of distractions. I wanted to spruce up the house a bit. I would be stuck more at home during recuperation and having more visitors. The addition of the TV we purchased recently, and the small decorating alterations it forced us to make in our den and living rooms had begun a series of improvements. I will simply say that I spent a great amount of time shopping and solving the easier problems in my life.

I heard from Laura today. It is likely that Art will need chemotherapy. They are constantly on my mind. My own experience tells me that there is comfort and power in gathering support and good wishes and prayers where and whenever possible.

Thursday, April 29, was my pre-surgical testing day. Vicki was still concerned about her cough and we all agreed John would bring me in for my appointment. As we traveled to the George Washington Bridge we heard a report that said an unauthorized car-carrier truck got stuck under Gracie Mansion closing down the entire highway for hours. John knew how to take an alternate route to where we needed to go, but that road was totally jammed. He decided the best course was to go to his office. From there he would lead us on foot to the subway. Then we could cross town and possibly arrive close to my appointment time. It was a very impressive plan and we arrived a mere ten minutes late.

He had originally planned to drop me off and go to work. I would call him later on when I completed my testing. Since the city was such a mess today, he asked the receptionist how long my appointment would take before deciding if he should leave me. She appeared certain it would take about forty-five minutes. A trip back and forth during that time seemed foolish to us both. In the end, it actually had taken more like two hours or more.

We started back via the subway to John's office. Hungry and tired somehow we managed to take the wrong train. John soon realized our situation and we got off to change directions. At this point we were running from one platform to another. All of a sudden I got some liquid in my eye. When I stopped in shock, I looked up only to see the filthy-fuzzy, black-grunge coated ceiling above me. It sickened me to think that anything dripped down and landed right in my eye from there. My God, if this cancer does not kill me, maybe this dangerous bacterium might. What the heck?

We kept going and soon decided to grab a fast lunch in the process. John brought me to a favorite office lunch spot. Frankly, it was not what I had in mind and I'm not that fussy.

I was reminded of something funny from our appointment. John made an unintended comment to the nurse-practitioner saying, "Amy is high-maintenance." He actually meant that I do *not* complain easily about medical issues; and that there can be problems I will not quickly bring to anyone's attention. He warned her to note that they might need a more "watchful eye" on me, because this is my general MO. Anyway, he used the wrong words and it got a little confusing there for a few minutes.

By the way, I know I am not a "high-maintenance" patient. I firmly believe that keeping my hairdresser and my medical professionals calm is in my best interest. Anyone with scissors, a knife or a needle in their hands is not the person I want to aggravate. I also don't want to complain and mislead the situation if I can avoid doing so. Perhaps, John has been witness to resulting delays to action in prior medical situations. I really understood why he tried to make his point, and it was funny how messed up it became. The nurse this morning probably thought we were both wacky.

It was now harder for me not to make comments such as: "Well, as long as I am high maintenance, next time can we have lunch somewhere else?" It was the second time he chose this food chain and neither time went well. Joking, I asked him where his co-worker had taken his wife who was also having medical problems. Actually, I was quite grateful that it was John who I went on this adventure with today. We stopped back at his office where his co-workers considerately showed concern about how I was doing. We were exhausted and left after a short time.

The next day was Friday—one week before my surgery. I made a last minute decision to go to the paint store. A plumbing problem in our main bathroom had taken a very long time to repair. We neglected to repaint the ceiling and wall to finish off that project. It seemed to me I could easily fix this before my second surgery. Painting is one of the few chores that I have been largely responsible for in the past. I am the better painter generally and John is better at preparing for the project.

Years ago, I had sponge painted the entire room. It was a quick fix to hide many problems the room has. This time I was sure that trying to duplicate color and texture would be impossible. My intention was to coordinate the job by introducing a stronger complimentary wall coloring. Friday afternoon and evening I prepared the room for the work to be quickly done the next day. There was a small amount of spackling and sanding to do prior to painting. That kind of work is not where I excel. After my best attempt I was ready to keep moving forward with the job. John and the girls thought I was silly, but they recognized that I was determined.

John had to work Saturday, as he often has to put in a sixth day. Knowing my plan, I think it was easier than usual for him to head off for an extra day.

I was confident it was a simple task to paint before picking Cara up from the S.A.T. test at noon. I worked easily applying two sponged coats. At first it was hard to decide, but the colors looked uncomplimentary to the room. I was disappointed and tired. After bringing Cara back home, she reluctantly shared my reaction to the poor color choices and I ran out to buy more paint. I came back with a much stronger color and finally, I was headed in the right direction. As the job progressed I thought about all the other things I wouldn't get to now, before my surgery on Friday. Later we all agreed that the room looked better.

Our friend called earlier in the morning, and asked if John and I would come by this evening for a quick pizza and an impromptu visit. Diane had not seen us since right before my mastectomy surgery. We had not been able to get together as she understood that my chemo treatments made me extremely cautious about everyone's health. For months it seemed like someone was not well. We all decided this was a good night to spend together.

I cleaned up after painting all day and looked forward to leaving our house. John needed the escape, too. He enjoys Diane's company as they both play guitar and he gets a kick out of her quirky humor. We all appreciated the time, and having a few laughs while several hours quickly flew by. I am glad we took advantage of the invitation.

I knew spending John's one day off on Sunday with the bathroom project was not a good idea. Looking at the room it occurred to me that I could take the remaining rose color paint and lighten it up a little. Then, I could apply that color to soften up the entire job just enough. John left for work Monday morning and I completed my project. It should have taken half the time, money and effort—what else is new. Now it is done, yay!

THE COUNTDOWN

T ime is slipping away. Anything else will have to be completed between Monday afternoon and Wednesday night. Thursday is surgery prep day. That means a clear liquid diet and a bottle of bowel-removal liquid that needs to start in the morning, which leaves you attached to the bathroom for the day.

Surgery was still at some unknown time on Friday. All this meant that the food shop and banking errands would have to be done on Wednesday. Also one more visit to Garry would be inserted into that day.

Monday's exhaustion from painting hit me. Hopes of spending time with Ginny before her ten-day vacation were quickly slipping away. We wished each other well and knew we would see each other on the other side of our respective plans. It seems that I have to make the most of cleaning the house on Tuesday. My biggest problem was I was feeling totally unnerved about this second event and it was coming up faster than I had imagined.

Tuesday was fairly productive. Not as many large cleaning jobs got taken care of, which was easier to let go of than most anxieties are.

Wednesday I managed my errands and a short visit to Garry. He had not been aware that he had a doctor's appointment that afternoon. His manager did not mention this appointment earlier, when she asked me if I could bring all the residents milk shakes. When I finally arrived, Garry had only a few minutes before they loaded him in the van to go for his appointment. I felt badly that this was such a short visit.

Mom and Irwin arrived from visiting mom's sister right after me. They also did not know of his appointment. Preferring more time with Garry today I would have skipped the ice-cream treats this time. I won't see my brother again for next few weeks, so we will phone each other often.

When I came home I wrote out a number of cards I had wanted to send out for Mother's Day and for various other reasons. I mailed them that evening so they would be delivered on time or earlier. It seemed like I was as ready as possible. I had spoken to a number of friends and family knowing the next time would be post-surgery before doing so again.

Thursday morning, I woke up with a small rash in my cleavage area. I had noticed itching there throughout my painting project. It was now pronounced enough so that I delayed the prep liquid and called the doctor's office at 9:00 to ask about what to do regarding this new development. They asked me to come in to New York for the doctor to determine if the operation should continue as scheduled or not.

Vicki and I ran to see the plastic surgeon. He was fairly confident that this was not a problem and thought it was a heat rash. Next, we saw a dermatologist on his floor to be more certain about the diagnosis. That doctor looked about seventeen years old. She evaluated the condition as "irritated sweat glands," which is basically another way of saying, it was heat rash. She also agreed that surgery was no problem for tomorrow.

One amusing moment of this day happened on our way home from the two doctors' offices. At several different junctures throughout the day, Vicki mentioned how unbearably hungry she was. I was quick to point out that I had eaten nothing and was not able to have anything until later tomorrow. I was getting a bit ornery. My sister was too hungry to be more considerate. We barked at each other several times. Finally she remarked, "I would be much nastier; however, I don't want to read about it in your journal someday!" We had a good laugh over that comment. Truthfully, it is something to keep in mind. Ha!

At this point, we did not get home until almost 4:00 in the afternoon. My prep had to start immediately. I had nothing to eat or drink all day. My concern was this preparation was started too late. The hospital representative who called to let me know surgery was scheduled for 7:00 am, told me not to worry and to continue the prep. She added, "Stay on only a clear liquid diet today. NO eating or drinking past midnight tonight."

Finally, I did the prep; I drank it quickly. It was not a pleasant experience, but I did my best. Yuck!

I used the topical cream the dermatologist prescribed for the rash before the first of two surgical soap showers. John and I woke up at 3:30 in the morning to be picked up by my sister at 4:30. Admission was at 5:45. Cara would go to school and Anne was going "to hold down the fort."

My overnight case contained a deck of cards, loose clothes, a pillow for the ride home and some snacks: four biscotti and a bag of fruit and nut mix to keep John and Vicki a slight bit more comfortable in an emergency. By that I mean a hunger-emergency, of course. It seemed to me that I was prepared and considerate, even at this time. What a gal!

SECOND SURGERY

May 7, 2010 finally arrived. Once again, my husband and sister came with me. It was not very long before the nurse called me and the whole process of surgery day began. It went quickly as I was the first operation of the day. I remember there were the usual introductions in the OR; I watched as my plastic surgeon prepared to start his day.

I was soon in a deep sleep. The next thing I recall was my husband, sister, and recovery nurse standing around me. Let me say this, I must be a true baseball fan. Even at this moment as I focused as clearly as I could manage I marveled at how much my male nurse looked like Tino Martinez, one of my all-time favorite Yankees. This young man was very nice and his southern accent was adorable. Was it the drugs? No, I believe Ron was a real cutie! This sounds like I felt better than I did.

Actually, I felt very much like a tree had fallen on me and I was not sure I had gotten free of it yet. My doctor decided I should spend one night in the hospital to recover. John and Vicki stepped out for a bite and met me back in my hospital room a while later. Slowly, I came out of my stupor and realized that an overnight arrangement sounded like the best idea of the day.

Also I remember two people, a man and a woman, wheeled me into my hospital room. I don't remember whether they were nurse and transport person, but that is my assumption. There they told me to move my hips slowly, moving from the recovery bed to the hospital room bed. After the implant exchange surgery and the five laparoscopic incisions made in my abdomen for the oophorectomy, this was a torturous request. They offered mostly verbal assistance, and though it was a struggle the task got accomplished.

Vicki and John spent a long time in my room napping uncomfortably in chairs. It became evident that it was a quiet, short-staffed weekend at the hospital. This staff seemed almost void of energy and interest. They did what they had to do without displaying much compassion or concern. The surgeons are hopefully great here, but generally the hospital staff is sorely lacking in people skills. A number of people have told me that scheduled surgery should not be done on Fridays, for just these same reasons.

My roommate had a tram surgery, the use of your own body tissue to build the breast after a mastectomy. She was in the hospital for over one-week already, due to additional issues. I believe her mastectomy had taken place some time ago. She was a beautiful black woman who had formerly worked at this hospital a number of years ago.

Obviously, there were problems between her and certain staff personnel. Before long and in between her visitors, there was a nasty altercation. My roommate read the riot act, big-time, to one of the nurses.

Throughout the rest of the night and morning hours she continued to voice her complaints in detail to anyone who entered her realm. Never during this time did we introduce ourselves. I was relieved for the curtain that separated our room. Since I did not want to hear her story, and I assumed she was less than interested in my presence, it seemed pointless to try and make conversation. There were implications that there might have been some racial aspect to the problem. Both John and I felt uncomfortable attempting an introduction that evening. Minding our own business seemed the prudent direction to stay in.

In the evening I had to use the bathroom and found it very difficult to get off the bed. The nurse had to unhook my pole from the equipment by my bed before I could drag the IV in the bathroom with me. Also, I had special electronic massaging pads wrapped around each of my lower legs to help prevent clots from forming. Before a trip to the bathroom or a walk these had to be unplugged and removed. This happened several times before breakfast the next morning. The anti-nausea medications worked great. I was relieved this experience was greatly improved from the one after my mastectomy

I remember that on the way back to bed the nurse stopped me to change the IV on the back of my left hand, and as she disconnected it the end of the line hit the floor. Vicki, who watches these activities extra carefully, was shocked as the nurse swabbed the line clean to return it to my hand. Vicki announced, "That definitely swiped the floor and it must be replaced." I could not have agreed more, and the nurse honored the request saying quietly, "I did clean it."

Later on, I awoke with severe neck and shoulder pains. I had to get out of bed as lying became unbearable. John remarked that I was pretty red in color about my face and neck. I was worried about having another allergic reaction like after the last surgery. When I went in the bathroom I was certain that this was definitely what was happening.

I used my buzzer and told the nurses' station that my skin color was turning red, and that it was likely another bad reaction to medication. The response came very, very slowly. Five minutes would have seemed reasonable, but this was much longer. Ultimately it took Vicki standing outside my room clapping her hands to get some attention. She said repeatedly, "We need some attention here." By this time, I was experiencing chest tightness like last time and shortness of breath, the latter of which I did not have last time, and I was scared!

Staff finally came in and said they called the doctor. They began to evaluate the situation. Before long I was placed on a heart monitor and oxygen. Again I received allergy medication. The doctor came and after a brief assessment ordered bloodwork to be drawn three times at intervals of eight hours to be sure I was not having heart issues. He was very calm and low key.

My roommate took advantage of his presence, and unloaded her saga on him as soon as he stepped in to see her as well. This doctor was a part of my plastic surgeon's covering team, though I did not realize that until later the next day.

After a time, the excitement quieted down substantially. Vicki agreed to leave John with me for the night and drove home. She would come back to drive us home whenever we were discharged. John was my hero. At this point I really felt mistrusting of being alone at the hospital. My husband was tired, cold, and uncomfortable both physically and emotionally. All he had was a blanket and a chair with foot stool. Though I never asked him to, he insisted on staying through the night.

Nighttime brought a small gaggle of medical staff, who all tried very hard to ingratiate themselves with my roommate. She had convinced them that she was a formidable adversary. It was obviously so; and it was interesting to see how she worked them over. It became pretty annoying as the conversations were loud and lengthy. If John were not there, it would have been impossible for me not to say something about the lack of consideration. Philosophies and cell numbers were shared, and some fences were possibly mended during the wee hours of the morning. I was more impressed by the lack of any courtesy by my roommate and her new fan club, than I was appreciative of the evening's efforts.

The next morning I decided that I would give one painless attempt to introduce us to my neighbor. As she stepped out of the bathroom and we made eye contact I asked, "How are you doing this morning?" She stepped toward us and we managed a brief conversation. She made some comments and suggestions. We were all cordial.

This woman looked about forty-five and was fully made up. She was quite stunning. Actually, we were shocked to find out later on that her oldest of three children was thirty-seven years old. She was off to the art room where she said, "I'm going to use a different part of my brain by painting a picture upside down." OK you go and have fun! Convinced this was helpful and good therapy she added, "This activity is more beneficial than sitting around feeling poorly and not receiving much help." Certain she was not going home for a while she already knew lots of ways to keep busy.

I told her that she looked great. She quickly pointed out that she would not do as I was doing and said, "You must never go without makeup, it's forbidden!" Also, she let me in on her own personal secret weapon by adding, "Get yourself a good wig and you will look great anytime." Listen, she was quite beautiful to begin with, and I am sure those were great pieces of advice. She also could be a bitch-on-wheels, so I was going to proceed with caution. We had a few benign and pleasant words during the next few hours.

By Saturday morning, I was still a bit reddish and blotchy, and my ankles, legs, feet and hands were fairly swollen. My tummy was mighty sore and whenever any movement was attempted it was horribly uncomfortable. I still had pain in my shoulder, which was likely the gas that collects after a laparoscopic procedure. The implants were much less of a bother. However, the drains under my arms were at best annoying. Blood was drawn a couple more times. That required bringing in the most competent person to handle my abused veins.

Walking was hampered by the fact that I had to keep my feet elevated due to swelling. It was evident that despite my general discomfort and awkward condition, it was time to work on being discharged.

The days of compassionate and advice-giving care is not easily found anymore. Of course, the staff was not completely inattentive. However, this care was discouraging and uninspiring. Perhaps better care is showered on the more "needy" individuals with more interesting or serious cases? I hope so. My double procedure and subsequent bad reaction to some medication and general post-surgery condition did not impress anyone here.

Yes, there have been lots of changes in the amount of staff due to cut-backs. Additionally, insurance companies and hospital policies require more paperwork than people-work gets done at hospitals now. How sad for us all.

Anyway, feeling poorly and nervous I still knew my best bet from today on was to get home. There, my family would be more helpful. Being at home would go a long way to making me feel much better. If I could manage to get comfortable enough I might actually catch some sleep. I left the hospital murmuring, "There's no place like home, there's no place like home."

My sister and Paul drove us home about 7:30 Saturday evening, May 8. There we found Anne and her boyfriend at home. Anne was making us hamburgers for a late dinner. That seemed like it might be a little heavy, but it was so sweet of her to have a plan. With my pink Yankees cap on to hide my surgery-bad-hair head, two drains bulging from under my clothes, no makeup and poor posture, I was a sight. Still, I was welcomed home and it was nice to be here.

Unfortunately, even with the painkillers, getting up frequently throughout the night hours became quite a task. The next day was Mother's Day and no matter what—I was glad to be home with my family. Usually we have been the hosts for this day. What a way to get out of that! Vicki, Paul and Jennifer had taken Mom and Irwin out for dinner. Mom and Irwin stopped by Garry's earlier, so everyone was taken care of.

Later on, the four of us ordered some Chinese food and Anne bought an ice cream cake for dessert to celebrate quietly. They gave me lovely cards and a pair of unusual earrings. Anne and I have had a "thing" about bees for a long time. I would find a stuffed animal bee or a bee card and write messages such as Bee Good, Bee Happy, Bee Wonderful, Bee the Best Person You Can Bee . . . and so on. Anne found little earrings with bees on them and wrote a lovely note with the Mom's Day card from all three children. It was lovely. Naturally the food choices caught up with me and I spent some time painfully, regretting my indulgences. It was very comforting for me to know that Anne was spending the week home with me again.

The next several days were rough, but not intolerable. The pain killers were an essential part of handling the situation; however, they come with a price. The constipation that is a side effect of the medications is awful. Combine that with discomfort from the gas remaining from the laparoscopic surgery and the pain from multiple incisions, and it was not fun. The drains were as annoying as I remembered. Include no showering and it was a pretty ugly affair. The plastic surgeon's nurse told me to come back on Thursday for a post-op visit and they would remove the drains. Wow, that sounded great.

Meanwhile, Anne was managing quite well to keep the laundry going, meals prepared, and general cleanup maintained. The weather was crummy and we did less walking than we had wanted to do. Tuesday, my brother-in-law Bob came by with some special instructions on how to get in and out of bed; tips from a guy with back issues are useful. After the first surgery, he had brought over a big foam wedge to use on my bed under the pillows. This was a big help again.

Diane also came by with a little lunch that she, Anne and I shared. It was thoughtful of her and the visit broke up our day nicely. A number of friends and family called to make sure I was doing OK and all wished me well. Garry called several times offering his concerns, too. Mom and Irwin left for their five-day trip to Colorado; they attended a graduation party for one grandson and a separate party another day celebrating the other grandson's recent wedding.

By Thursday, May 13, I was anxious to get into the city to have the drains removed. My early appointment went well. The nurse and doctor seemed happy with the way surgery went and easily removed the drains. The nurse gave me two special bras which must be worn day and night for six weeks. This impedes pockets of fluid that form and can cause problems. My rash was now spreading below my breasts towards my belly. It seemed like the surgical bra and drains might be aggravating the condition. A different bra might be helpful. I got home feeling more human already. After the next forty-eight hours I could take a shower. What a lovely thought, I just couldn't wait!

By Saturday evening, I showered knowing that when it was done I would be a new person. Sunday I wanted to wear makeup and get back to appearing more like myself again.

Mary and Bob came by for a short visit. It was good for us to have their company. Barbara and Tom stopped in later with lasagna for our dinner. They also were brief in their stay. Coincidentally, Loretta called and generously sent over sausage and macaroni, too. We left the lasagna for another day knowing it would be appreciated as much then, as on this particular night.

Food gifts are great as they provide such a treat for everyone. This second surgery is not creating the same stir as my first one last summer, but people have been just wonderful. Ginny managed a few text messages while away and called when she got home on Sunday afternoon.

Mom and Irwin had a very good time away and were back on Monday. Tuesday Ginny came by for a visit and we went for a little walk, which was just what I needed. Colette called again and reminded me that we spoke earlier last week after I came home from the hospital. It was very vague in my mind and indicative of how hazy I must have felt. She is going to come by soon, but not this week. Good, it is something to look forward to.

Diane came by with another lunch. She had brought me a ton of movies to watch last week. I returned some and she borrowed a few of ours in a swap. It will be fun to see how successful we are at picking out flicks for each other.

Wednesday was a quiet day which was used to catch up on my journaling. Garry called and reminded me that he missed me, saying, "I would love a visit anytime, and remember your friends are welcome to come, too." He thought my not driving shouldn't stop me from a visit; he is a character even now.

Between Anne and Ginny I have managed short errands to the bank and food store this week. That lets me feel there is a bit more "normalcy" to my world already. The laundry gets taken to the washer in handfuls as opposed to basketfuls and that is fine. Vacuuming was done once slowly, as compared with the usual three or four times this week and that's OK. The week slipped by calmly and uneventfully, which is all good.

John had his own doctor's appointment today and ended up at home for the rest of the day. Things are settling back down and into place again.

RECUPERATION OR SOMETHING LIKE IT

This last weekend was very quiet. John continued to make the most of the weather and time by tackling his list of household jobs. Keith came home as he needed temporary housing before his apartment is available this summer. He has been driving back and forth to a job he started on Monday.

Sunday Keith and I decided to head out to buy cases of water. First, I went for a short walk before we left to do our errand. The rest of the day I was tired and crashed on the couch in front of the TV.

Monday morning I went for a walk by myself and felt pretty good. Colette called earlier to tell me she could come by today. I knew it would be great to have her company. This no-driving business is not easy no matter how good or poorly I am feeling. My friend came by with homemade whole wheat banana bread. Mmmm dee-lish! She wanted me to save it to share with my family later. We sat at the kitchen table drinking coffee and talked away the afternoon.

Hey, I just realized that coffee is probably part of the reason I had such trouble sleeping last night. Coffee is an indulgence that I allow myself in the early morning hours occasionally. Big mistake, I got no sleep!

Today, Ginny and I went for a walk. We went up one moderate sized hill in my neighborhood extending the walk a little more today. My one side around the largest abdominal incision was a bit more sore and uncomfortable indicating that I might be overdoing things a bit. Mom and Irwin stopped over and the four of us stood on the driveway talking a while longer. By the time I came back inside, the walk and the heat had wiped me out.

Tomorrow, May 26, Vicki and I will go into the city where I have two doctor's appointments. My stomach is a little sore and my system is still messed up after I eat, which is particularly uncomfortable. It will be good to have the gynecological post-op visit to check out whether I am on track. Vicki and I haven't seen each other for almost two weeks. The last time was when I had the drains removed at the plastic surgeon's office. She has been busy, but manages to call most days to check up on me regardless of her schedule.

Those visits went well and were simply routine post-op appointments. The doctors assured me that everything was fine. We grabbed a light lunch in between appointments and were both anxious to return home afterward.

The month following my second breast surgery was less dramatic than the last summer's event. Anne continued to be a big help. John was pitching in by accompanying me on many of the tasks I usually take care of by myself. Cara was helpful with a moderate amount of housework.

Cara was finishing up her sophomore year and gearing up for theater camp, which was to start two days before the last day of school. We hadn't realized that timing when we signed up for the first session. This was an unusual Christmas present from my cousin Peter and his wife Carol. Lucky girl! We all agreed this would be a fantastic opportunity.

At this point though, I was becoming concerned about all the details. The idea of Cara going away for three weeks was becoming a reality and it was starting to worry me. I knew how exciting this was going to be for her, but it was a difficult step for me. These plans made me even more anxious to get back to driving and a more normal life again.

The doctor had told me not to drive for approximately four weeks, and definitely not while still taking pain killers. About four weeks after surgery I knew it was fine for me to start driving again. It was great to be independent and I was being careful; although I was probably running around more than was ideal.

It was also important to get back to visiting Garry. I missed him and was concerned because he had stopped calling me about two weeks earlier. Physically handling his phone had become impossible for him. It was evident his body was rapidly deteriorating.

We had been informed in early June that Garry's place of work needed to arrange for his last day to be planned. Also he was going to be moved out of the group home, where he had lived for almost twelve years. He would be moved to another group home; this second home was for more severely limited people. The hope was that it would have more appropriate care thereby eliminating the necessity of a nursing home for him.

All of this was going to be so tough for my brother to accept. He will be leaving his job that he loves and the home where he was so comfortable. He has grown attached to so many people in both places. We are all so worried about how Garry will handle all these adjustments.

Mom, Irwin and I were able to check out the new group home where he will be transferred to. It seemed like a more wheelchair-accessible home. However, it wasn't as homey and it felt more like a care facility. The other residents were of such extreme limitations that there would be no ability to make any connections with them. I knew from conversations with my brother he was fearful of going to a nursing home; the only selling point here was that this was another group home. As both group homes are owned by the same organization, Garry was already familiar with some of the staff and residents.

Much to my own surprise, *I* found this move horribly upsetting. At one point I broke down in tears as the new manager spoke to us about bringing Garry into this second home. His social worker joined us. She planned to leave us to meet Garry and to tell him of the plan. I insisted on being included on this. We met outside my brother's home and nervously stepped inside.

Garry listened carefully. He seemed more heartbroken about saying goodbye to his job of the past twenty-eight years than anything else he had to accept so far.

He tried to credit everyone at his workplace and the staff at his home with taking great care of him. He expressed that he really did not think these changes were necessary. We all had to remind him that his condition had become more serious and there was no longer any other choice. He was told by everyone how much he would be missed. We also promised him he would be visited by and could keep in touch with his many acquaintances and friends.

Garry asked me to come and see his workplace before he left the job. At last he had convinced me to meet the people that I had heard about for so many years and see his office for myself.

The social worker told my brother an opening at a better equipped group home for people who were more physically limited was now available. This move would take place in a few days. This meant his job would also end on Monday of the coming week; it was a real one-two punch!

It was important to me that I was there with Garry. This was one of the saddest experiences for me personally. I wanted to reassure him that our family would be by his side all the way. I thought he should know that we all agreed that these changes could not be put off any longer. I knew that his coworkers and his present home-staff had done more than we could have asked them to do. He absolutely understood they did their best to accommodate his situation for a long time.

Honestly, I think we expected that Garry might not last before these changes were made. My plan was to continue my own recovery and do whatever it took to help my brother, Mom and Irwin.

As I promised, I met him Monday, June 14, at his job on the last morning. It was touching to see him at his desk as he encouraged his replacement. Garry had been the receptionist and official greeter at this office. It was obvious that he could no longer perform his duties. He was seated in the area watching all those who came by. He spoke to anyone who was kind enough to engage him in a word or two. Mostly, he would fall asleep for brief periods of time. Going to work every day was a great source of pride and it had given him a sense of purpose. His job was his lifeline and we knew this change was going to crush him.

This rehabilitation center provides services for mentally challenged adults and a workshop that employs them. As weak and upset as he was today, Garry wanted me to meet his work buddies and see the whole place. After a short time, I had a good glimpse of how dearly beloved he is by them. His desk had many photos on it as I expected. It embarrassed me that through all the years, this was my only visit here.

Everyone was very caring and it was clearly a sad parting for all. After a time, I left too "chicken" to stay to the very end. I was gratified to see the workplace that he loved so dearly. He was proud that he had been awarded the plaque last December, which recognized him as the dedicated and valued employee he had been. Mom and Irwin arrived sometime after I left. Since a number of key people were on vacation a retirement party would take place in about a month. In my mind it was doubtful this plan would happen, but not for lack of good intentions.

Next was the actual move to the second group home. It was under ten minutes from our home to this new residence. Garry was annoyed about sharing a bedroom with another fellow. My brother has always had his own room and this idea did not sit well. His roommate could not communicate and continually made sounds. In fact, none of the persons who lived here functioned on even a moderate level. Garry is physically a wreck, but he is mentally as sharp as ever. Making matters worse, my brother is having trouble keeping food and liquids down and chokes frequently.

Mom, Irwin and the rest of our family all visited Garry throughout the week. I made sure to take Cara by to see her uncle before she left for camp. As always he was glad to see her. It was terrible to see how much the quality of his life was continuing to decline. It was a neat and clean house, but it didn't feel like he had a home anymore.

My efforts were split as Cara was leaving on Sunday for camp. It was not easy, but we managed to stay focused. Some of the shopping we did together, but I picked up as much as I could on my own while Cara was in school. She is a pretty easy spirit and quite undemanding. I think she is excited and a bit nervous about leaving. Auditions will be held during the first couple of days, which does not help with the anticipated jitters.

Cara's friends had a little send-off party for her Saturday night. It felt more like she would be gone for three months than for three weeks. With all the commotion of the past week's running around my recuperation period had come to an end. There were more important things going on that required my focus and attention.

John and I were going to get a glimpse of what it feels like to be "empty nesters." I was thinking about how much quieter things were bound to be, and that we would get a break from chauffeuring duties. I was trying to remain calm, but everyone knew that I was a wreck about my daughter going away for the next few weeks.

THINGS GOT CRAZIER

onday morning, June 21, we were ready to take Cara to camp. It seemed imperative to me that we make the effort to arrive early. In my most negative frame of mind, I pictured us getting lost and making a last-minute entry into a room where all the girls had already bonded, leaving Cara "out in the cold." To add to my imaginary poor start, I was sure Cara would be stuck with the one bed that no one wanted for some horrible reason. It was a total anxiety attack. Cara was ready and anxious to get started.

We arrived at Stagedoor Manor camp in the Catskills in less than two hours. We were definitely among the early arrivers. The camp was swarming with theater geeks of all ages and sizes—mostly the staff at that point. They all had outrageous costumes and full makeup on and were extremely friendly. It felt a bit goofy.

We followed instructions and got Cara settled in and registered. She was the first to get to her room and the choice of beds was hers. She picked the bottom bunk bed next to the window. This was a fine choice. The rooms were unattractive at best. Obviously, this was also my first camp experience. There were six beds and six dressers in a long room with one bathroom to be shared. Ah, that was a challenge to be sure; six female teens and one bathroom. How does that work? Well, I imagine some compromises are ahead.

Cara was very anxious to meet her roommates. Yet, no one came for a very long time. We could hear lots of other people running around, and we were starting to feel left out. We went on a tour and kept checking back to the room. Finally, the others came and we could see Cara was in her element and ready for us to leave. Two of her roommates were returning campers who were excited to see each other again. One girl was from Puerto Rico and another one from Scotland, among the other roommates. Everything seemed OK.

We left certain this was going to be an impactful experience and wonderful opportunity. The camp had taken all cell phones away on our arrival. They were not to be given back to the campers until next Sunday. It was going to be torturous not to talk to our daughter for a week. I couldn't wait to pick her up already!

I had driven up to camp while John navigated the trip. It was more of a strain than I thought and left me especially sore under my arms. All in all, the day had gone well. We expected to be a little more carefree for the next few weeks, because our schedules often revolve around Cara's plans. Actually, the twenty-day camp required our attendance by day eighteen. So, this time was relatively short. As I fell off to sleep, I wondered how comfortable my baby was and if she missed us, too? Hah, hah!

The very first day started with an early phone call from my mother. Garry had been taken to the hospital because he could not keep anything down and was dehydrated. I met Mom and Irwin there. Truthfully, it was a relief to see Garry in this environment. He was surrounded by friendly and attentive medical staff. He seemed much more comfortable and happier.

My brother requested this hospital because he knew that my friend works there. She actually works in maternity. Laura has a particular fondness for Garry and managed to visit him throughout her work week. By the week's end, we found out that he had an acid reflux condition complicating his other issues.

The doctor spoke about my brother's deteriorating condition caused by the ALS, and mentioned that a feeding tube may be needed. We collectively decided against that measure. The hospital contacted the nursing home we wanted most to hear from; they agreed to take Garry temporarily to recuperate.

In just a couple of short weeks Garry had lived in two homes, and spent a week in the hospital. He left his job of twenty-eight years, and also moved into a nursing home. It was all very unsettling. We were praying that he would be able to stay at this nursing home for the rest of his life. However, at this time we did not know if that was possible. The expected move would take place in a couple of days.

This same week another crisis occurred. Anne called me to see if she could talk to me before I left to see Garry at the hospital for the day. I recognized her extremely-upset voice and told her to come home right away.

When she arrived with her boyfriend, I could see she was totally distraught. She became hysterical telling me about the events of her morning: Anne had gone to work as usual at the bank. After a short time she went out on a break to get a bagel for herself and another employee. She stopped at a convenience store she was familiar with to cash in a scratch-off lottery ticket first. The man running the store was a bank customer she knew for almost two years. He came in front of his counter by her and pushed her against the wall. He proceeded to touch her inappropriately and said disgusting things to her. Shocked and scared, she blurted out, "They know where I am and will come looking for me if I don't get back quickly!" He let her leave without further struggle.

When she went back to work in tears no one knew what to do for her. They also did not know what to make of their customer's behavior, and were probably stunned by the story. They told her she could go home because she couldn't calm down. Anne was surprised that they were not more protective and compassionate in their responses. Making things more awkward was that one co-worker was a personal acquaintance of this man and his family.

Then, Anne went to her boyfriends' house where she has been living and showered and changed her clothes, as the smell of the man's chewing tobacco was still with her. She was so distraught that Dave and his mom convinced her to talk to me next. I was incensed by the account and insisted on her telling the police about the incident right away.

We ended up at the police station all afternoon. It was very tough for Anne. We all agreed this person should be stopped from any similar future actions. Charges were filed though we knew that there was no evidence to lead to any certain end. Our hopes were that he might plead guilty to a lesser charge, which would create a record. Then, any subsequent charges would have more serious consequences.

What a day! What a week! What a year! We left certain this event was the beginning of another enormous problem. The charge was "sexual contact" considered the least of the sexual offense charges. After a few difficult hours, we already understood why these and worse sexual offenses are rarely reported. This all seemed unreal!

My mom had called in the midst of our day to find out when I was meeting them. I told her Anne was fine, but at the Police Station with me, which I would explain when I got to the hospital. I was too exhausted to even begin to think of how to hide what was going on. At this point, we all had such serious things to deal with that keeping secrets did not feel right.

My friend Diane surprised me and had been waiting at the hospital with Garry and my parents. When I explained what had happened they were all shocked by the details of the day.

A couple of days later, Garry was moved to the nursing home where we wanted him to be. There he seemed to be slightly more content than he was at the second group home. It was probably because he had his own room again. We tried to bring in some things to personalize this space, and make him feel more at home. All of us are uncomfortable knowing that the caregivers don't know him at all here. His communication is poor even on a good day and he is almost visibly mistrusting.

The frustration and anger Garry displays does not give a clue to his real character. These people are not likely going to know what a wonderful and loving person he has always been. They won't know that they are meeting one of the kindest human beings ever. How sad!

It was easier for me to spend many hours with Garry, Mom and Irwin while Cara was away. This allowed us opportunities to speak to the caregivers we met throughout the week. We explained my brother's condition, his needs, and his preferences as best we could.

The amount of visitors and cards were incredibly heartwarming. Like at his group homes, this was a kosher facility. Garry was not a fan of the food or the dietary restrictions, which he manages to complain about. He also did not make any attempt to win over the Rabbi who stopped by to make his introduction.

Actually my brother had been required to attend services and make appropriate religious observances through his group home. He had been fine with all that except for one very bad experience a few years ago. The group home went to services and afterward ate at the Temple's offering to the community—a small number of insensitive persons complained that they did not feel the group home residents should help themselves to the food provided at the table. This seemed like a particularly inappropriate place to encounter such treatment; leaving Garry with some reluctance and discomfort for what part religion should have in his life. Now, isn't likely the time that the nursing home's Rabbi will become a trusted friend.

My brother's reflux issues are a huge problem and therefore it is necessary to restrict his soda consumption. Garry has been a Coca-Cola addict for years and this limitation adds greatly to his misery. We did the best to help him adjust. We understood there were too many changes especially in the past one-and-a-half years. No one would be able to go through this ordeal without fear and frustration.

We hung the photo collages I had made and some of his awards. We placed photo albums, balloons, and joke books around the room.

Of course, we managed to display a few Coca-Cola memorabilia as well. Everywhere he looked we wanted to remind him how special he has been. I cannot be positive what my brother thinks, feels, or expects anymore.

We wanted the staff to be able to see how important and special Garry was. This was a person who had friends of every color, shape, size, gender, age and background. He would compliment people generously and even bring out the best in those normally impervious to such attempts. How could these people possibly guess what a terrific guy he had always been? They couldn't.

Here is a perfect example: A few years ago, he told a disheveled cashier that she looked very pretty as he checked out of a store with my mother. Later Mom asked him, "Didn't you notice how dirty and unattractive that person was? Why would you give her such a compliment?" Mom was slightly annoyed at a certain lack of sincerity and discretion on his part. Garry's reply made her feel almost ashamed that she had questioned the intention. He said, "Of course I did. But, I thought she probably doesn't hear many compliments and she might like to get one, too." This was Garry.

I have an awful feeling that we have all been somewhat dishonest with him. With each move we told him he would have better and more appropriate care. In truth, each move has made him feel less secure and unhappier in most regards.

Other than visiting my brother, I still have my medical appointments and normal daily tasks and concerns. Keith started his first Monday thru Friday, nine-to-five job working for a small computer company. We were glad he was among the lucky few to have a job this summer. This will be great experience to have on his resume. He seemed to be off to a good start and our fingers are crossed. Keith also has summer classes four nights a week and a knee surgery this summer.

Cara had finally phoned sounding very enthusiastic about camp and we were thrilled to hear from her. She will be performing in *"Avenue Q."* She described it as hilarious and sometimes inappropriate *Sesame Street*. I was not sure what to make of that? Anyway, she sounded wonderful.

She requested me to send down some snacks as the camp's food was not up to home-standards. Also, Cara asked John to copy a piece of music for her to use in a class she was taking. By the next day, I sent a big box. It also included a note and the music. I made sure there was plenty to share and offered a wide variety: cookies, candy, nuts and pretzels. There were lots of little packs to avoid big open bags of food. What a huge hit! I received big thanks for the thoughtful, prompt response.

We missed Cara and we were about halfway through her time away already. John and I had taken advantage of this by going out to eat frequently, which is unusual for us. That helped me as I was busy spending extra time with Garry each day.

I had told Colette that I would go with her to see her mom at her nursing home in Pennsylvania soon. I wanted to do this while Cara was away. Being far away for a day would be easier right now. Our general sense of security has been rocked since Anne went to the police and reported the incident involving the store operator. Perhaps we were somewhat paranoid. Bringing charges against an individual is not an easy thing to do. I told Cara's friends to stay out of that particular store saying only, "I've heard he is not a good person." I did not want them to know more for now; I had not explained to Cara what was going on and did not want her to worry. This was her fun time.

I went to visit Colette's mom on July 6. I had known her almost my whole life. We lived right across the street from each other and I was constantly in their home.

Colette's mom is deaf, which is why she ended up living in this particular nursing home two hours away from her daughter. The distance was a trade-off for her being able to communicate with her caregivers, who all used sign language. There were other accommodations making it the best decision. Etta, of course, might not always agree as she missed more frequent company. Colette is devoted to her mother and has taken care of her about seven years now. First, there was in-house care. When it became impossible for that to continue, this nursing home was the next step in a very difficult process. Colette faithfully visits at least one day a week.

As I anticipated, her mom was glad to see me. She inquired about my whole family. She expressed real concern for my mom and my brother. She is wheelchair bound; having the use of only one hand and poor eye sight due to cataracts. The quality of her life has been compromised. Etta said, "I just want to go home." I could see how much Colette's company consoled her, but there was little joy in her expression. It is all pretty awful, this sick and old stuff.

I was glad to spend the time with my former neighbor and to make the trip with my friend. My mom has sent Etta notes, which have been sincerely appreciated. Colette's mom would love more contact from outside and is very lonely; we all wish she was living closer.

—⁂—

Our family went by Tom and Barbara's for July 4. They have become the official hosts and it was pleasant and quiet. They did most of the work. Again, we tried our best to share what we could.

John and I were looking forward to the next weekend, when we were going to the Catskills for two nights. We will see the performance weekend shows. We never get away so even this tiny trip was exciting. I had waited a little too long and reservations were not easily made. I had two choices. Knowing we were spending most of the time at camp I decided to save some money. That was a big mistake, but I will get to that shortly.

I gave Garry an early birthday present a few days before we left to get Cara again. He had recently mentioned he had always hoped to find a shirt that said "flirt" on it. He only wears short sleeved t-shirts and prefers them to have funny sayings, slogans, or be from meaningful places. I had a Coca-Cola red shirt made up with "flirt" and a large-white number "1" placed on the front and "GARRY" on the back. His eyes widened and I knew he loved it.

Needed Breaks

J uly 10, was Garry's birthday; however, we had to see Cara's performances, and bring her home from camp. We felt awful about not being with him, but there was no choice. John and I arrived at camp and met up with our daughter quickly. It was obvious she was having a great time. We were introduced to a few people, who were all rushing off to wherever they needed to be.

Cara was in two performances. The shows that the camp put on in less than three weeks time were absolutely amazing. I think there were a total of fourteen performances. The talent of most of these young actors just blew us away. This was fantastic fun!

Cara's show was a total blast and the score was silly and riotously funny! Cara surprised us by starting the show as the focal point dressed in a large sun costume, her face coming out the hole in the center. She was wearing the biggest happy face ever. Cara did a tap dance, and though dancing is not in her comfort zone, it was adorable.

The rest of the time, she was on stage in the ensemble dressed as a policewoman. She had no speaking lines and just enjoyed being involved in the production. She sang and moved about while we delighted in watching every moment.

My cousins were not only generous to send Cara to camp; they also made the trip to see this performance. It was terrific sharing the success of their gift. Their youngest son spent many years at this very same camp and this brought back numerous good memories for them. Afterward we grabbed Cara and the five of us went out for dinner. Peter and Carol picked the restaurant being somewhat familiar with the area. We had a lovely meal and all things definitely *not* being equal we treated them to say "thanks." I was glad we had a little time apart from the usual big family gatherings with my cousins. They seemed equally pleased that Cara had a wonderful experience as they fully expected.

John, Cara and I went back to the camp to see different shows the rest of the evening. It was amazing to see such talent. We were in awe of all the hard work that goes into these successful efforts. Then we said goodnight to Cara and went to our motel.

Our accommodations were like something out of the *Shining* or some other horror flick. We got out of our car reluctantly, as there was a strange group of people hanging around outside. When we got to the desk the personnel seemed unprofessional and rather creepy. The woman at the desk handed me a can of spray disinfectant and our room card-key. She explained that the only room left was a "smoking room" and we might need to use the spray. Oy. We knew this was going to be special.

The whole place was moldy smelling, and not well maintained. Our room was on ground level, it had a terribly noisy air conditioner, the rug was not well vacuumed, and the blanket very gnarly. The smoke was the least of the issues here. There was also sliding glass doors to the outside making us feel even less secure. Holy shitoly, we were skeeved out!

Our night there was not what we had hoped for. I followed John's lead and covered my pillow with the shirt I had worn during the day. I brought the sheet over me, but made sure not to bring the cover up to touch my skin. We barely slept as there were so many weird sounds. I knew that the area was booked up because of camp weekend and a church retreat that was going on as well. We hurried out the next day and did not look forward to returning for the second night.

We had breakfast without Cara, as we had not heard from her and assumed that her time would be tied up with the commotion of the day. Just as we left the diner, she called wanting us to take her out for a bite. We snatched her up and took her for a quick breakfast at the local coffee shop as time was running short.

We went back to camp and enjoyed taking in the rest of the day. Anne, Dave, Cara's friend and her dad came to Cara's evening performance. They all loved the show. Luckily the threatening storm held off until the tented show ended.

John and I saw more performances indoors even later into the night. Cara was obligated to join in certain activities, so we were on our own. Before leaving performance weekend we managed to see part or all of six different shows. We spoke to some of the other parents as we made our way around. In the course of conversation we discovered our motel had a well-known bad reputation. We drew many laughs when we announced where we were staying.

The evening was tremendous fun, despite knowing we were headed back to our motel. We were so tired that falling asleep was easier then on the first night. However, we awoke at 7:00 to our next door neighbor yelling at his ex-wife on his phone. By their conversation's end, we knew far too much about this anonymous person. What a crazy place! We left as quickly as we could.

The camp asked everyone to pick up their campers early to go home. Cara has surely made a few friends that she will continue to keep in touch with for a long time. She was proud and joyful. It had turned out to be a fabulous experience. Still, Cara was looking forward to catching up with hometown friends, and was anxious to indulge in her own home's amenities. John and I felt similarly regarding the latter. We were all happy for the adventure.

My cousins want Cara to decide if she would like to go to camp again next summer. She had not assumed this offer would be extended for a second time. It should have seemed like a no-brainer, but Cara explained next summer should be extremely busy. She was thinking ahead to college plans starting, a summer job, and driving practice for a driver's test in early next August. Oh, boy, next summer is a runaway train already! It impressed me that she had these considerations on her almost-16-years-old mind.

I was beyond thrilled about how this all worked out for our daughter. We were delighted to have her back home again; and all three of us slept soundly in our own comfy beds!

CATCHING UP

All the craziness of recent months left me with little time to journal. I worked on my project less as I found myself getting more overwhelmed by Garry's situation. I was also sinking into the after-surgery and recovery "blahs." I found it difficult to find time to write. I did jot down plenty of notes to remind me of certain details. These will be used from this point on to catch up with my journal.

John, Cara and I missed Garry's 55th birthday while we were at camp. It was a bad day for Garry, who was in too much discomfort. He barely was able to spend a good moment with any of his company. The plan to have cake and his visitors in a small private room had been unrealistic. Vicki, Paul and Jen were there along with others. Everyone was upset by his condition.

About a week later Irwin's son Alan, his wife Kathy and their youngest son came from Colorado to visit. They wanted to try and help our parents. Garry was considerably better and was pleased to see them. The weather allowed for some nice time on the attractive patio outside the home. Alan and Kathy's son also has special needs, and knowing Garry has been a significant inspiration for them.

In the meantime, I was bringing Laura and Colette to see Garry for visits that they wanted to make. My friends, Diane and Ginny, have been thoughtfully sending notes and cards he enjoys. I couldn't ask or expect more of any of them.

My brother has so many wonderful friends and acquaintances. He has had sporadic visits by his co-workers and by his first group home residents and staff. Those have been very special and naturally, also difficult. All these people are helping him to realize how much he is loved and missed by those who are so important to him. I can hardly believe how many people Garry has impacted through the years.

John and I have joked about the comparatively small handful of people that would be at either of our sides if circumstances were reversed. John says he would have to pay people for sure. *It makes one think about being a better, kinder and gentler person.*

Vicki and I barely connected and I missed her company, but she was trying to keep her business together. It was getting busier than it had been in a long time. She was having some medical issues of her own and the various stresses were taking a toll on her. My sister knew that I was available to help our mom, and it was one area she needed to have me step up to right now. We all continued to do whatever we had to do.

Cara's birthday, on August 4, was a small event. Her friends were vacationing and I decided to take two of her buddies to breakfast before they left. After that, they had the rest of the day together. We decided to have a home-BBQ party in a couple of weeks to better mark the occasion. Cara had been to a number of sweet sixteen bashes and she understood it was not possible for us to have one of those. She thought a low-key gathering prior to school starting again would be fine.

Planning her party was hampered by Keith's scheduled surgery, on August 16. Gee, last year I came home from my first surgery on this day. This year we were taking Keith for surgery. That day is also John and my thirty-fifth wedding anniversary, which seemed relatively unimportant. Oh my, Cara's birthday would wait.

It was hard to deal with all these other things while continuing to be consumed by my brother's issues and needs. Knowing you don't get another chance to do some things later on, we were trying to balance this all as best we could. Life does go on.

Cara started her driving lessons after her birthday and now is driving on a permit. I have been trying to take her out often before school starts again, when the time is harder to find. I am trying very hard to be calm and more patient. Anne and Keith have often described me as "bad" at this job. Cara has less confidence than they exhibited and I am afraid to discourage her.

John spoke with his sister Rita, who mentioned that our nephew Dan and a small group of his friends were putting on their own musical production at a tiny theater near them. We said we would come out to see his show on Saturday night. John, Keith, Cara, and I went to see the show which was fun. We were glad to be supportive and it presented us a brief opportunity to see Rita and her children.

We had a huge laugh at Rita's expense that I have to mention. It will surely remain in the Dempsey folklore: While following her to the performance in our car, we pointed out several of Rita's driving mistakes to Cara. You know like: "Notice, Aunt Rita is driving too fast . . . Aunt Rita is making an illegal turn . . . Aunt Rita doesn't have her signal on, and . . . Oops, Aunt Rita just ran over all the geese crossing the road!"

The last one created a huge feather cloud that engulfed her truck. After the initial shock we immediately started to roar with laughter. Yes, that story is true and a keeper! Driving Lesson 101 was over. It sounds terrible, but it was so awful that it was funny!

ANNIVERSARIES
AND SPECIAL DAYS

A couple of days before our wedding anniversary I passed a real milestone: August 14, 2010, was the one year anniversary of my mastectomy. *This was big.* There was no party. It was merely a fact shared a couple of times throughout the course of the day. Even though it was a non-celebrated event, I felt the seriousness of how important keeping count would become as time passed.

In some ways it was hard to believe all that I have been through in this one year. It's shocking, really! It is becoming more apparent to me that I'm feeling the impact more since my second surgery. Perhaps, that is because it is more clear to me what effect my decisions have had on me.

At some point I may join a support group. I would probably have done that by now, if other circumstances were not absorbing my time. Admittedly, I had felt certain and confident that outside support was not needed last year. My sister, my neighbor, and my school friend are each inspirations. Their stories are different, as none of them went the same route. Still I do wish there were even better options for being proactive. Yes, it could be much worse.

I had a follow-up appointment with my plastic surgeon. He found everything to be fine. I voiced my concerns about sleep difficulties and described being disturbed while lying on my sides because of discomfort, which inevitably awakens me.

The doctor explained, "Everyone is different. Some heal with little remaining discomfort; while other patients are not as lucky." Adding to that, "Some people take a little longer—give it another six months. By then, you should be healed pretty much as well as you will be." He was emphatic that my discomfort was due to the healing process from the mastectomy. Though, probably more right than wrong, *he* has never had implants. This doctor had one piece of advice: "Don't focus on the discomfort or pain. If you do, it will never go away." Even while trying to appreciate what he was telling me I wanted to kick him! My sister and I were not impressed by this display of compassion. We left and headed for home.

—ᴍ—

My visits are as frequent as possible to Garry. It is harder to spend big chunks of the day with him, but I go very often. Now that Cara was home there were many other things going on. She and I try to practice driving almost every day. It seemed important to me that we should spend some fun time, too. We managed to catch a couple of movies and went out shopping a bit. With Keith's knee operation coming up quickly, we were trying to squeeze in as much as we could. The next week would be donated to his needs.

Keith had taken on finding the doctor and scheduling the surgery himself. Now, John and I were feeling pretty anxious about the surgery details. We would have still felt this way even if we had been more involved.

I called the doctor's office and spoke to the nurse. I asked her what should be expected post-surgery. The nurse was honest and to the point. She strongly suggested that he come back home, where he would need a lot of help for one or two weeks. He would be in substantial pain requiring pain killers and he would not be driving for six weeks. So, we were bracing for additional concerns, extra help for him and more worries, for *me,* as John and Keith are not worriers.

The best thing happened to Garry this week. The nursing home's music-activities person has been trying to encourage him to join in some of the scheduled events that are available. She is a lovely, energetic woman about my age. Garry has flatly refused to take her up on any invitations though she comes to see him almost daily. We try to encourage him as well. He loves music, especially familiar songs that he can sing along with. After many weeks, he decided to try the music hour with Mom and Irwin accompanying him. This woman actually plays the piano there. He knew and sang many of the songs. Though he can barely talk he sang his heart out.

Garry said it was his best day there. He would look forward to the Monday scheduled hour from now on. Mom and Irwin were thrilled it went so well.

The music gal was glowing with the rewards of her success. She and my brother are now "friends." This dedicated woman made a convert out of him. I think she will help spread the word that he is really a good fellow; despite his new-found love for cursing at the staff. This seemed like a real breakthrough. Just knowing he is able to have some pleasure now makes us all feel a little better.

Anne and Dave came by on Sunday to wish Keith good luck. I subtly mentioned something about the date and the fact that it was our thirty-fifth anniversary on the next day. Anne was a little embarrassed and admitted with everything else she had forgotten this one. I was of course giving her a hard time and I wasn't upset at all. There was definitely too much going on. They left and returned a little while later with a card and cake. We enjoyed the dessert with them. As always, Anne provided the mini-celebration.

Monday, August 16, the day of Keith's surgery arrived. We got out at 3:30 in the morning to get Keith to a hospital located near his college by 5:30. We were all nervous. The nurses and doctors were very reassuring and appeared qualified.

Keith went off to the operating room after a short time and we went to the waiting area. We would get word from the doctor when it was over and Keith was sent to recovery. Thank goodness John had taken the day off, as I would have been a wreck by myself. We were wrecks together. All went better than expected. The doctor called after a three-hour procedure and reported all was fine. He did not think that a second surgery on the knee would be needed as was originally suspected. The doctor was able to reattach Keith's hamstring, and wanted to see him in one week; physical therapy would start weeks later.

Uncle Bob's pillow-wedge came to the rescue once again. Everything was set up as best as we could manage. Keith was not as mobile as he had expected, and the pain was intense. He needed the pain killers as frequently as allowed. Except for getting up to go to the bathroom, he stayed in bed and used the equipment as instructed religiously. He was a good patient and we were glad he had come home.

Unfortunately, I came down with a fever and a sore throat on Thursday evening. By this time, Keith was feeling better able to manage his own situation. I must say I had given him the best care for four days. By Sunday, he decided to have us take him back to his apartment. He wanted to go back to work Monday. I was not in agreement, but he insisted on this plan. Keith arranged to have a friend drive him to work and to his doctors' appointments for a while.

John and I tried to settle him in as best we could at his apartment. The place was an awful mess and I was uncomfortable about the whole idea. We cleaned up a bit and lectured a lot. It was not the mess that sent me over the edge. But, since our presence was expected it might have been wiser that he cleaned up before surgery; he certainly won't be doing much of that for a while. OMG r u 4real! I was overruled from the beginning and so we left him to fend for himself, which he does quite well.

The good news was that Keith was anxious to go back to work. Keith did not want to miss another paycheck and it was his last week to work full-time for a while. This, I considered a good sign. School would start the week after this. Oh my goodness, how would he be able to get around the campus so soon? On crutches, obviously! I tried telling myself he would gain much from this experience. It would force him to work harder than ever. Keith will have four days of classes, two full work days, recuperation, and eventually, physical therapy on his plate for this, his senior year's first semester.

With Keith back in his apartment, we returned to our usual activities again. We decided to make quick plans for Cara's birthday BBQ on this Saturday. Before we knew it we had things under control. I got busy making all the food. We had lots of extras and a delicious chocolate birthday cake and cookies. The guests ate, laughed and talked non-stop for hours. It all worked out fine. They stayed outside until deciding to walk to the park around the corner for a while. When they left I stepped out on the deck to clean up. They had been thoughtful and already had taken on that job. Wow, they really are growing up. They returned about an hour later, wanting to come inside to get away from the bugs. Everyone appeared to be happy. I think Cara was pleased as it was just enough of an event. Aunt Mary and Uncle Bob came by just in time for some cake and kept John and I company for a while.

The next day we had plenty of leftovers and with a few additions we invited Grandma, Grandpa, Anne, Dave, Vicki and Paul for dinner. Since Grandpa was turning eighty-nine years old the next day we got a birthday apple pie for him. We already had leftover birthday cake.

It was even more of a low-key celebration than Cara's party. Mom and Irwin were not expecting or wanting much in terms of celebrating. We were all feeling fairly worn out from everything that has been going on for a long time now. It may have been an inadequate way to mark either Cara or Irwin's birthdays, with these small get-togethers. Garry, Jennifer and Keith were all missing this one and we did the best we could.

Labor Day weekend I noticed my bug bite from the last weekend had gotten weird. I ended up at the emergency room where a doctor told me it was infected and she prescribed a topical cream. I used the cream for several days. When no improvement occurred I went to my GP with concern about Lyme or West Nile. Thinking it was more likely an infected spider bite he prescribed a different cream.

Coincidentally, I had been on two different antibiotics recently; one which I was just finishing. The medicine was for the strangest sore throat I had on and off for six weeks. The first antibiotic did nothing. The second medication I had taken a month later seemed to work well. Oddly enough this was actually good medicine for a problem bug-bite.

Between the sore throat, the bug bite and the additional random itching I went to my doctor three times in three weeks. The third time he insisted on a long and serious talk with me. He told me that stress can actually cause physical issues and he thought this was what might be going on with me. I was surprised to have him speak to me this way. He continued by telling me, "Anyone facing serious medical problems can become stressed out and manifest all kinds of symptoms."

My doctor suggested I try to cope better and de-stress through exercise, extended faith practice, confiding in a close person, or a new outlet. Yeah, I got what he was saying . . . But, I did not bite myself in the leg, I *did* have a horrible sore throat on and off for six weeks and I was itchy as all get out! I was sure a new hobby was not the entire answer.

Actually, I was not upset by anything he said. So, surprise, surprise I am stressed to the max. What else is new? He gave me a prescription for a light "chill pill." When I filled the order at my pharmacy I spoke with the pharmacist. He quickly looked up my records and said with confidence that the itch was a common reaction to the second antibiotic I had taken. He suggested I try a dose or two of allergy medication, and see what happens. I did that and by the next day, the itch was gone. Maybe everyone was a little right.

Labor Day, was guess where? Yep, Tom and Barbara did the hosting job again. They included John's Aunt Betty, whom we had not seen in a long time. I felt terrible that since my diagnosis and Garry's situation, I have had almost no time with her. I do feel like I have been somewhat selfish recently. I hope she understands and knows it is not a reflection of my feelings for her. We were delighted to see her and she seemed to enjoy the day as well.

I went to see Garry the next day and found nothing terribly new. He luckily has had a hospice-aide five days a week. He gets shaved every couple of days and a couple or more ice-cream cups each day with her extra attention. Otherwise, he is not happy about her. The aide is supposed to spend two hours a day with him. In reality she stays about forty-five minutes and literally disappears. My mom is afraid to complain because she is content knowing that the aide feeds Garry lunch and cleans him up a bit. All he will eat is soup and ice-cream. Basically, we think nothing will help him feel more comfortable.

My brother tells me, "Go home." whenever he does not agree with what I say to him. I cannot stand the way he treats the staff and I give him mini-lectures about that. Garry was never unkind to people and rarely if ever cursed, *ever*. Sometimes, I leave relieved to have been rudely dismissed. I return in a day or two hoping he will be more pleasant.

At times my brother is calm and content with company. He listens to his favorite old TV shows in the background. Some days he sits in his special hospital-chair outside on the patio area with us and seems fairly content to be out in the fresh air.

Vicki and I hardly see each other anymore. Our phone calls are less frequent now, but we do text brief updates. I am frustrated by the change in our relationship these past six months. She can be very secretive and private for someone who can be right up your . . . ! My sister has the ability to withdraw from family drama and stress when she personally feels the ill effects of such times. She is also a control freak, and there is no control in Garry's case.

Vicki tries to be positive as much as possible and so, all this is maybe even less tolerable for her. Mom and I are much more negative. Mom and I usually expect the worst. It is just too much on any of us, and sharing the responsibility as much as we can does help.

Vicki has not been going to my doctor appointments with me lately. Fortunately, Anne has been able to drive me to New York on her days off.

John and I managed to meet Vicki and Paul over the weekend for dinner. It was nice to have this relaxation time with the four of us. Paul's birthday the next day, September 11, made us being together even more appropriate. Just saying that date still makes me sad, and this made noting his birthday one day ahead easier.

Keith started school and was calling often with updates. He was managing to do all that he needs to do. Naturally he is anxious to get back to driving. Getting around on crutches was definitely a "pain in the . . . leg." He still cannot put his full weight on his leg and it does still hurt. Both the doctor and physical therapist think he is doing very well so far. His class load is heavy, and this is going to be a tough semester. Keith also mentioned he is going to help manage his rugby team and handle their website. Perhaps I should stop worrying about him? Yeah, OK!

Cara started her junior year. She was unhappy about summer being over. It was depressing for us all. We have been robbed of much of the fun and relaxation time that the season could offer, particularly these past couple of years.

September is an adjustment month to be sure. This being eleventh grade, we knew it was going to be a challenging year. Everyone starts to focus on college much more seriously. It makes me weak in the knees to even say it. As always, she is anxiously waiting to find out about our school play. That will be where her energy will be directed once practices are a part of her schedule again.

One nice occasion came about in September. My mom's old friends, Joan and Marvin, were celebrating their sixtieth wedding anniversary. They have invited Mom, Irwin, Vicki, Paul, John and me to come to their party. We have seen them infrequently in recent years, and it sounded like it would be a wonderful event.

Joan and my mom became friends when Joan's son and Garry were in a special education pre-school program together about fifty years ago. Our families went away together a couple of times when I was young and my father was still alive. John and I actually worked for them at a restaurant and bar they co-owned with other friends at the Jersey shore one summer while John was still in college.

Mom and Irwin have kept the friendship going. Since Joan and Marvin moved to Pennsylvania, the two couples don't see much of one another. The invitation came at a very difficult time for our family. Had Garry been healthy he would have been included. My mother was extremely uncomfortable about leaving him for the day. The rest of us knew it was a much-needed diversion and wanted to plan on attending the party.

Grandma asked Anne to spend the party afternoon with Uncle Garry. Anne was fine about this plan and ended up enlisting Dave and Cara to join her. My mother was now on board for the event.

The invitation stated "your presence is your present." We decided that a small group gift would be fun anyway. After we took care of that, we each included our own cards. I also decided to write a letter with some of my memories of spending time with their family. Joan is a big fan of my annual Christmas letter and I thought she would like this. In addition, I typed up a list of "Some of the Most Famous Couples" to which I added their names.

Assembling the gift provided a bit of a distraction from the stress of going back and forth to the nursing home.

We were so pleased to have been able to join our friends and to see their sons, who were now men with grown children of their own. In truth, the party had given each of us a lift. The break was especially good for my mother. She looked so much better and happier the following week; it was great to see the transformation in her even for a little while.

SUMMER ENDS
AND ALL CONTINUES

My mother, more than anyone else, was in a terrible position. Her baby was going through such a horrendous ordeal. He had issues since birth and had been her extra "special" lifelong concern. She and Irwin have spent every day with Garry for months, staying with him for many hours each time. It is increasingly difficult for her to leave his care and management to others. As fine a facility as he is in, there is never enough attention for your loved one.

Garry's extreme physical limitations make everything more difficult. Knowing that he is mentally functioning and trapped in this totally deteriorated condition is intolerable. His body is unmanageably frozen and he is in constant discomfort from lack of changing positions. His reflux issue and choking have forced him to stop eating ice-cream his only luxury and indulgence. Garry also cannot have soda which is critical to him, as this was his exclusive choice of liquids.

Sometimes, we see his old sweet personality. More and more he is disengaged and annoyed. We want to be with him and yet, it is very difficult at the same time.

Irwin is usually good with Garry, but the one's bad hearing and the other's poor speech are a difficult combination. Some days it is a strain for Irwin to stay as long as mom wants. Irwin is generally active and a sports fan; Garry hates to watch any sports activity on TV. Occasionally, Irwin has an anxiety attack if my mother is not willing to leave the nursing home when he is ready. All this can be unnerving on top of what is already awful. This was one of those days and I left as soon as it was not good for me to be there longer.

Colette and I have been talking often and compare nursing home woes. Her visits with my family have been sweet and comforting.

Laura is one of Garry's "faves" and always brings out some of his best efforts. She is very comfortable with him and will touch him by rubbing his arm or giving him a big hug. It is easy to sense how much security he finds in her company. She tells him, "I miss all your jokes and compliments. But, even a little smile from you is so wonderful!"

After we leave, she gets a little tearful and then she composes herself quickly and tells me she will be back very soon. This is the way each of her visits goes. Her husband Art is having a tougher time on chemo than I did, but we hope that he will also make out well. It is incredible that with everything else going on in her life, Laura finds time for us. I have special friends who were there for me through my cancer crisis and continue to be there for Garry and my family.

Though I have needed the exercise and companionship, my walking has been put aside. My time with Ginny has been limited by our schedules. We manage to talk and I hope we will get back to encouraging each other soon.

Carol from high school finally wrote again. I was relieved to hear that she had been away on a long visit with her daughter's family. She seemed great and that was all I needed to know. I wrote her back immediately.

We saw our friends Maryann and Tony spontaneously. We don't make enough effort to see others and to do things. The more I talk to people, the more I think lots of other people are the same way. Most of the time, it helps to enjoy a little variation in your activity and have some good company to share it with. Otherwise, you lose it!

Anne was notified by the court-appointed attorney today that there is a scheduled court hearing in the County Courthouse in two days. The attorney suggested that we come to the court hearing on Thursday, where we could ask questions of her and see for ourselves what was going on.

It was not possible for John to take the day off. I went to court with Anne and Dave. Wow! Court provided us with an eye-opening experience as this judge was hearing all sexual related cases. It is shocking to have even a glimpse of what is happening around you every day.

Our attorney finally came in and found us. We stepped outside into the hall where she explained that she was already informed that the man who had groped Anne was going to plead "not guilty" today. If the judge were to do anything to this man, who was a first-time offender, he would be offered a Pre-Trial Intervention, or PTI. He would have to comply with the program for a time of one to three years as set by the judge. After he completed the program, there would be no record of any offense and that would be all.

Instead, our attorney was going to ask the judge to send the case back to the municipality where the offense occurred. She felt that there would be a greater vested interest in how the store owner/operators conduct themselves inside their own town. This seemed to make more sense. It is possible that there he might plead "guilty" to a lesser offence, which would create a record on him.

As there were no witnesses the chances of a conviction are slim. Of course, this forum will mean Anne will likely have to testify. Uncomfortable and difficult for her, she is committed to seeing this through. Her actions are really admirable, and we hope it will help her in the end. We left knowing this was not over.

I had not heard from Colette since she let me know that her mom's cataract procedure had been performed last Tuesday. I decided to text my friend just to get an update Monday morning. Unfortunately, her mother had a mild heart attack since we spoke. Having already had heart procedures and a stroke in recent years this was worrisome.

Etta was upset and wanted her daughter to stay with her for several days. My heart went out to them both. Like my brother, her mom has a body that is failing her and a sharp mind. I know about some of what Colette is going through, as she agonizes over the best ways for her to support and care for her loved one. A day or two later, the emergency was over and I was glad to hear that my friend was finally home again.

I remember how John was with me overnight the last time I was at the hospital. I recalled how anxious he was to leave the hospital the next day. It is not easy to deal with these emergencies.

Meeting the Music Man

O ne morning I arrived earlier than usual to see Garry. As he was not awake or ready for breakfast; I decided to get a cup of coffee from the café. It was a lovely summer morning and I thought to sit quietly outside on the patio. A resident was sitting in his wheelchair and playing an old cassette player.

I sipped my coffee and found the music completely relaxing. Nat King Cole was serenading us. After a while I got up and as I passed the man I told him how much I liked his music. He had a pleasant smile and a twinkle in his eye and responded, "I'm glad that you enjoyed the music."

Days later, Mom and Irwin had gone to visit her sister Betty. I went to see Garry early with the plan to stay awhile. He wanted to sit outside. Again I saw the same man listening to his music. He had all the old crooners and some Big Band sounds playing today. I went to sit at the next table hoping Garry would be able to hear better from there.

Acknowledging the man I said, "Good morning, we are going to sit close by and listen to your wonderful music. I hope you don't mind?" To that he replied, "Please, come sit right here and listen." Unsure about this plan, but not wanting to be rude, we moved to his table. As it turned out it was a pleasure to talk to this gentle, sweet man. His name is Alex and he has been in the home a year-and-a-half now. His wife was at the nursing home first and she has passed away. Alex explained his son-in-law had been an early contributor to the nursing home, "So, it was easier for me to get in."

This is a highly regarded facility and we feel Garry was very lucky to be placed here. Maybe it is another case of divine intervention? All that can be said in any event is: *Thank You! Thank You! Thank You!*

I also found out that Alex was from the Bronx. Wow, my folks are also from there. I wanted to introduce him to them. Alex told me that he had just come from a reading of someone's memoir which included stories about the Catskills, from years ago. He had the best time listening as it brought back great memories of his own. Now I knew he had to meet Mom and Irwin as they too had been there often in earlier years.

Garry listened to the music and sang a little to the few selections he recognized. I could tell my brother was content and comfortable. Alex seemed happy to have our company, and we sat talking and listened for over an hour until he was ready to go inside.

Mom and Irwin surprised me by coming back from their trip with my Aunt Betty (as opposed to John's Aunt Betty). Betty had not seen my brother since her husband's memorial service last summer. Garry was really pleased to see his aunt again and smiled. We were all glad for the opportunity to be together this afternoon.

It was days before I saw Alex outside again. This time I brought a couple of old cassette tapes I had. They had Nat King Cole, Johnny Mathis and Barry Manilow on them and I hoped my new acquaintance might appreciate adding them to his extensive collection. Alex seemed pleased at the gesture. When I reminded him that I wanted to introduce him to my folks he insisted that now would be a fine time. So, I waved them to come right over to us.

As I expected, this was an easy and valued introduction. Instantly names and places were recalled and Mom, Irwin and Alex were becoming fast, new-old friends. Irwin is eighty-nine years old and Alex is, too. They knew so many of the same people from the Bronx. As they remembered their names Alex would smile and Irwin would get teary eyed. They laughed and were ecstatic to meet each other and share these memories.

Mom couldn't believe that Alex and she had gone to the same grammar school and delighted in stories about the Catskills. This was really a special encounter, which brought me such pleasure to be a part of it happening. It was a boost for Irwin especially, to have this new friend here and it seemed to mean as much to Alex. Later Alex happily told the Rabbi, "I finally found another eighty-nine-year-old who responds that I can talk with!"

It is apparent to me from knowing Colette's mom, Alex and my brother's situations that it is easy for others not to recognize how sharp their minds are, because of the conditions that leave them in wheelchairs. They are three very different people with different stories. I am aware in Etta and Garry's cases that people are shocked at how clear-minded they are. Alex is able to communicate easily, but when I used to see him planted in his spot listening to his music he often sat with his head hanging from having nodded off. I did not guess that he was as "sharp as a tack." *Our assumptions when incorrect can rob people of their well-earned dignity.*

With little intention, I found this incredibly intelligent and engaging person. It is obvious that the majority of people in the nursing home are in bad shape in some way or other. It saddens me though to think of the ones who are still able to make connections and are not able to find people to ease their loneliness.

Meeting Alex has been a treat, as he still seems filled with joy despite any physical problems. Much of his time is spent corresponding with people. He relishes his memories and lights up when he talks about his family. He loves and enjoys his wonderful music! This was by far the nicest thing to have happened here for quite a while.

FALL MOVES IN

There was a surprise at the nursing home today. Upon my arrival I discovered my brother was upset and in the process of moving to a new room. Mom was also a bit disturbed by the plan to put him upstairs in the "long term" part of the home. She knows each new adjustment is unwelcomed by Garry.

A hospice RN told us this service might be coming to an end. Garry would not mind that at all; as far as he was concerned he was only interested in my mom's help. My mom, however, was starting to panic. Garry was already angered having been just told again, that he was going to have to totally give up his soda and ice cream. These eliminations were made based on the frequent choking fits that plagued him. The medical consensus was that they may aggravate his acid reflux problem and create even more choking issues.

All I could think was that I wanted him to have some little pleasure in his existence. It seems to me that the ALS caused the deterioration of his swallowing and probably also the coughing. I don't think "what" he eats is the main problem. Of course, I'm no expert. He has always had an atrocious diet, but to deny him these small indulgences now feels cruel to me. While I may be wrong, I want to give him the ice cream and soda and the heck with it! It is understandable that the staff does not want to encourage anything that might be causing additional issues. Their job is to care *for* him—I care *about* him. We are all concerned about him choking.

My brother must weigh about eighty pounds; just the skin and bones of his scant five-foot frame are left. Garry literally is incapable of doing one thing for himself. Speaking barely comes and mostly goes. What he is able to communicate tells us that his mind is intact. He will turn his head slightly to one side in the direction to look to someone he cannot see. In his usually weakened-alert state his "yes" and "no" answers are difficult to distinguish at times. There is a slight rise and fall to his eyebrows and sometimes cheek with his "yes" that gives a hint to his actual reply.

Mom, Irwin, our social worker and I moved most of the things from the walls and counter tops. Aides brought the rest of my brother's things up on a dolly. We made quick order of the room and the switch was completed. Though it is the same furniture and nearly the identical space, we carried on about how there was something much nicer about this new room. Truthfully, there were a number of nails and tacks on the walls in just the right places and Garry's picture collages and awards fit perfectly here.

Garry was not buying the whole deal. He was completely unhappy today. Imagine how suspicious he is becoming with all the changes in his life of the past two years, especially those since mid-June? We don't think he expects to die soon. He only expresses some current pain complaints regarding his physical condition. This is heartbreaking.

It was a particularly tough week as Garry seemed not to be making the adjustment well. Thank goodness Laura came to visit on Friday. Garry had remarked long ago to me, "Laura is one of the best things you have ever done." Then he added, "For me too!" Hmmm, how many ways can he get me? It came out funny when he said it and it still strikes me that way. As always, her presence helped. He considers her another sister. She's the good one.

Next, there is a confession of sorts that needs to be made. Laura smuggled in something for Garry to eat. Although she was aware the home was kosher she hoped Garry would be allowed to eat something non-kosher in his own room. Before leaving at her last visit, she asked if there was something Garry wanted her to bring next time. He replied, "Something to eat." She did not want to disappoint him. This is a serious rule to break. It is a fundamental law at this home that no food or drink is brought from the outside that is not approved first. We were not only breaking the home's law we were breaking—THE LAW.

It brought a broad smile to Garry's face as he saw the cup of rice pudding come out of her pocketbook. The three of us were defiant and reckless and it felt good! He was thrilled with the contraband. Though we were terribly nervous, we laughed about our success. It was the best thing that happened all week. I did not want to get my brother in trouble, but I did not think God would *really* mind and that's what counted.

Saturday John and I were in bad need of a break. John had been after me for some time to find out when and where we could go and hear a couple of our former high school classmates' band. I was less enthusiastic, as it was a little scary to think of running into people we had not seen in years.

We went to a local bar and restaurant to hear them that evening. They were in a five-piece band that played old early rock tunes. There were many familiar, and many not-so-familiar-anymore people who were there from our youth. This was a refreshing change of pace. I especially enjoyed catching up with an old grammar school friend who had lived right around the corner from me. We spoke to some people more that night than I remember ever doing before; everyone seemed to enjoy themselves.

Oddly, the very next morning we received a random call from another high school friend we hadn't seen in years. He and his wife had come from Pennsylvania to help his mother return home from the hospital.

After a bit of arranging, the plan was that John would head over to meet him at a local spot. I would swing by separately for a short time and then go to see my brother as I had planned earlier.

I could have skipped my visit to Garry, but I try to keep my word. As I arrived late my visit was not very long. Mom and Irwin left shortly after I came by. Then, Vicki and Paul stopped in after me and I chose to leave them to a private visit. It is easier to say goodbye when my brother is not left alone.

Anne took me to my breast surgeon's follow-up appointment today, Oct 7. I must go every six months for the first two years, after which those appointments will be once every year. The doctor's assistant came in first. We talked at length and she was very supportive. After she left my doctor came in to examine me as well. We spoke about my discomforts and sleep issues. She did agree with most of what my plastic surgeon had said and yet, she thought that over time there might be even more improvement. This doctor thought that not sleeping well *is* a large issue and said she could give me a sleep-aide if I want to give that a try. I will think it over for now. I still have not tried the "chill pill" either, as dependency issues are another concern.

Anne and I had a rare day alone together. She was great about driving in the city and giving up her day off. Whenever she works Saturday at the bank, she gets another day off during the week. It's still an imposition, and I appreciate her loving support. First, we had a bite to eat as we were early. It provided us time for a long talk. I got caught up on what she is up to lately. Then I bought a pink ribbon pin for myself and a pink support wrist band for Anne at the hospital gift shop. The appointment was quicker than usual and we were back home by 3:00.

It is terrible that I haven't gotten the hang of this trip, or the determination to be independent of anyone's help in this regard. City driving really frightens me. It may be soon that I should find some courage and a good GPS. However, today was fine.

By the way, I haven't mentioned very much about my Yankees. This was not my favorite baseball season. Even so, I watch most of the games faithfully. I am somewhat surprised and happy to report that they have already won Games 1 and 2 of this year's playoff games; despite my doubting their chances of going all the way. Go, Yanks!

The rest of the week went by quietly and uneventfully. Garry seems to be in declining spirits in general. I went for two walks with Ginny. We brought each other up to speed; these times together always cheer me up.

John stayed at home on Friday as there were all kinds of household problems that required his attention. He needed to work on Saturday again this week, and so he decided to take this day. He did manage to break away from the tasks here and joined me to see my brother. Garry was glad to see him. John enjoyed the many photos in the room and brought some to our attention which helped pass the time. After a while Garry started to choke a lot and I knew John had enough for this visit. We left Garry with Mom and Irwin.

John went to work on Saturday. Later on, the door opened and I was surprised by Keith. It was great to see him! It had actually been almost seven weeks since his surgery. He just got back to driving recently and this was his first opportunity to come home. He was so busy that I didn't even know when he might be able to make this happen. We sat and talked for some time while we anxiously waited to surprise John. Upon seeing Keith's car outside John came in, happy to see his long-lost son.

After a short time Keith joined Cara and me for a driving lesson. He was very curious how *that* was going. She was less into the activity than we were and it was decided to be enough for this day.

Keith wanted a little rest time at home and that was what he got. He was happy to have a TV that was hooked up to "cable" to see whatever he wanted to watch again. My son watched football in one room and I watched baseball in another. Occasionally, John checked in with both games. We were happy to have Keith home—even if it seems like a terrible way of showing it.

John spent more time with baseball as it was Game 3 of the playoffs. It was great as the Yankees swept the Twins in three. Yay, Yanks! Now there would not be another Yankee game until Friday. Hopefully, they will rest up enough so that they will be ready for the job.

Monday was Columbus Day and Cara had off from school. She had lots of homework, but wanted to go to Garry's for a short visit and a driving lesson as well. It was a break from studying. We stayed just long enough and until he seemed too uncomfortable to enjoy even his niece's company.

Tuesday morning Ginny and I met for a walk. Our commitment to this exercise has been poor. With my need to visit Garry often and to be available to pick Cara up from school it is tough to manage the time. As it is, my day in between those two activities can be filled with errands and cleaning and cooking. Ginny is very productive with her time and is always busy. Her children are all older and on their own. While she is very involved in their lives, it is still not the same as having a child at home in public school.

Wednesday afternoon Colette called and filled me in on her mom's condition. Colette was a bit anxiety ridden with the events of the last two weeks. My heart really goes out to her for what *they* are dealing with. She plans to visit more with her mom over the next week. We are hopeful to get together possibly later next week. It was good to talk with her and of course, she was also interested in how Garry is doing.

Today, I went to see my brother as the weather may be awful tomorrow. Garry was pretty good for a while with Vicki, Jen, Mom, Irwin and me having come at about the same time. We all went to the café. It was a different atmosphere for my brother and we could grab some lunch. He demanded we go back upstairs after a short time.

Jen had to leave to catch a bus back to the city. I was glad to see both my sister and niece. I said goodbye to Garry when his hospice aide arrived, as I hate to hear him complain and get angry at her. She is the fourth and best one he has had. Hopefully, she will stay a while despite his current lack of graces and charm. Sadly, those were always two of his strongest qualities.

Alex was coming our way just as I was leaving. Mom, Irwin and I walked down the hall to meet him while Garry was being cleaned up by the hospice aide. I was happy to spend some time with our newest friend. Every time we talk I get to know him a little better. He is a definite favorite of the home. Everyone knows him by name and he knows all of them, too.

The next day, Laura called to say she was going to try and visit Garry despite some heavy rain. Later it became obvious she would be too late. She would have come minutes before his hospice person. Garry would be nasty to the aide for interfering with Laura's time with him. I felt badly but thought it best to discourage this visit. We will try again next week.

By 2:30 I received a call from my mother wanting to know where we were; I thought I had made it clear that we *might* be there today. I could hear the discomfort as Mom already told Garry we were coming. There was nothing to be done now. That is why I do not tell him in advance about visitors. I felt badly for this unintentional disappointment.

This was a tough week: Colette's mom's was not well, our brother-in-law Bob's mom was very sick, and John's Aunt Betty had news that her son-in-law was in the hospital, too. We are keeping them all in our thoughts.

Keith came home again Friday evening. John and I were watching the Yankees' first American League Championship Series game. He must have brought some good luck with him. What started to look like a disaster for the Yanks, turned around in the seventh inning and ended up to be a huge win over the Rangers. From now on, Keith will have to watch the rest of their games. It's the baseball "superstition thing." We need all the help we can get!

Saturday afternoon John, Keith and I went for a visit to my brother. Garry always asks about Keith and had not seen him in quite a while. These visits are not easy for Keith, who manages fine with his Uncle Garry, yet is fairly reluctant to plan a visit. It was important and I felt much better that they saw each other. My brother had other company making it a little easier than some visits. We all told stories to pass the time more pleasantly. Grandma and Grandpa were thrilled to also see Keith again.

Later that evening we settled in to watch more baseball. This time the Yanks lost. I am really having a hard time expecting them to pull this series off. Great, now it is *my* fault if they lose.

Keith and I took Cara out for another driving lesson. We overdid it and after lots of dual instruction, Cara got pretty upset with the both of us. It would be easier if she was enjoying it more and I am trying my best to be reasonable with her. Everyone knows I am a "horrible back seat driver." Oh, brother!

Mary called with news that Bob's mom had passed away. She was ninety-six and has been in failing health for a long time. Our family got to know her best when she would stay with Mary and Bob around the holidays. They would stop over at our home to celebrate a post-Christmas Day and we always enjoyed her joining us. We will attend the funeral later this week.

Meanwhile the Yanks came home to lose both Games 3 and 4. Our pitching was not doing the job and the bats were not making up for it, which was disappointing. Laura has also been following the game more this year. That may have to do with the fact that our friend Jane's nephew was drafted into the Yankees' organization this past spring. We are all so excited for him, and are eager to watch his future unfold. He is in their AA League, how cool is that?

Laura came late Tuesday morning to go with me to see Garry. He seemed quieter than usual with us. We left as his aide arrived. We told him Laura had to leave to make an afternoon work meeting. It was not the truth; it spared us all his anger at our leaving.

On the way out Laura and I stopped by to see the belly dancer who was going to perform in the activity room for the patients today. We waited for a long time and laughed at how unusually popular this show was. The residents were early and anxious for the show to begin. Finally, we decided not to make the highlight of *our* week about the belly dancer at the nursing home. It may have been a mistake though as Irwin, Alex and Mom thought she was great. Garry had gone into his bed already and missed this entirely. It is always good to find something that makes you smile, which obviously can be found anywhere.

Wednesday evening John, Cara and I headed to Bob's mother's wake. As we were stuck in the worst traffic, it turned into a two-and-a-quarter hour trip. The game was on the radio in the car and the Yanks won! That made traffic issues much more tolerable.

Cara wanted to pay her respects, but was slightly uncomfortable about going to the wake. We talked about what a "good" and long life Mae had. I was confident that everyone would be handling it well. Truthfully, I thought it was the right thing to do, and beneficial for Cara to have more experience with this type of event. It may be harder to deal with this part of life when you do *not* have a strong religious foundation. The lack of certain beliefs can make death seem more strange and difficult to accept.

For me, I find my thoughts on death change as I get older, and have different experiences and relationships. My hopes are that there is a place where those who have earned it find rewards and peace. It was not until after my father died that I realized my belief in God. What I believe about that entity is still vague and often confusing. I feel spiritual and not religious. I'm not personally big on coming back. I do believe that I feel people who have passed out of my life are sometimes present in some form. I am a fan of "signs" and miracles. The idea of angels among us is acceptable and welcomed. This all might not make me the best example of a Jew—yet, honestly I mean no disrespect. I accept all good people and good deeds and good thoughts as the "right way." Jeepers, I'm getting too preachy. Hey, it is my journal!

—w—

The next morning, Tom, Barbara and Anne joined John and me to drive down to the funeral. It was a lovely service in a beautiful, huge, stone church. We then went to the cemetery. Later we joined Bob's family at a luncheon following the ceremony. It was a long day and I was pleased that Anne wanted to be with us to pay her respects. She is very responsible in these matters and I know Mary and Bob were pleased.

When we got home Anne found a notice in the mail box concerning a court date for the municipal hearing regarding her case. It was scheduled for two weeks from now. We were surprised at how soon it would take place. The lawyer had thought it would be much further away. I could see Anne wishing she had not received this news yet.

Friday, I went to see Garry about 1:00. Today I was a little freer with the time. John was going out with his co-workers as one of them was moving to England. Cara was going out to a friend's house after school; I was not needed for a ride home until later at night.

Garry and I ended up having a long and exceptionally good visit. Mom and Irwin had to leave earlier than usual. I was glad to be able to be with my brother. He was difficult to understand, yet more energetic today and thus he tried harder to repeat himself. He actually told me, "I'm so happy to see you today." The statement almost shocked me! I told him, "Garry that's the nicest thing you've ever said to me—I feel like a superstar!" He just smiled. He always saves his big compliments for persons other than Mom, Vicki, or I. So this acknowledgment meant so much to me, really!

We talked about our dad, my children, our family, Garry's loyal friends, his need to be nicer to the staff here, his TV programs and so on. All went well until after I fed him his dinner, after which he began to cough and choke. Garry was not resigned to me leaving as he knew no one else was at my home. I waited a while and got an aide to check his oxygen level. When he was settled down, I explained that I had stayed longer than I expected and was going to have to leave. He asked me why? I explained that I was hungry, in need of doing some household jobs, and planning to watch the ball game.

Garry has become very demanding about his limited needs. He often seems annoyed about what he considers to be our late arrivals, and even more about our early departures. In other words, our days for him are never long enough. Finally, he dismissed me and I knew he was slightly disappointed that he could not persuade me to stay even longer. I went home exhausted and satisfied. October 21, was a very good day.

Just as I settled in to watch Game 6 my phone rang. It was Diane, who wanted to stop over with a plate of brownies for me. These were for my birthday on Sunday. She did not want to intrude by barging over. I explained that I was alone and she was welcome to watch with me. When she came over we talked through at least five innings. The game was terrible, but I was glad to see my friend again.

We said goodbye when Cara and her friends called for me to pick them up across town. I was not happy about their timing as I knew the game was almost over. Even though this loss was clear, I like to see the entire game, especially such an important one. Texas has never won this title and I knew it would be a big deal for them.

I felt that the girls should have called earlier or waited until the game was over. Still I did the job; they were aware that I was annoyed and seemed somewhat amused.

John had come home from his night just when I picked up the girls. He does not have any interest in any of the game hoopla so he changed the channel. After returning home I went into the back room and continued watching the post-game show. My family felt my disapproval and they were not particularly happy with me, either. We all got over it and that ended the season. Life goes on—after all, it *is* only a game!

The next day John took me out to do some birthday shopping. We decided to buy a GPS. It was exciting for me as I have a terrible sense of direction, and I do not enjoy driving to unfamiliar destinations. Hopefully, this will be a big help. Everyone seems to find these devices to be an asset. Great!

Vicki called and invited John and I to dinner later Saturday evening. We met them at a local Italian restaurant. It was great to spend some relaxing time together. My birthday is also the anniversary of Vicki's twenty-fourth year as a breast cancer survivor. We toasted to her continued success, as well as mine. We are sisters in more ways than one!

My birthday brought some cards and calls from close friends and family. Keith called with his greeting and apologized for his absence. It was fine, as I understood and was glad to have had him home the last two weekends. Cara and I went to see Garry for a short visit. I thought he would be happier if we had some birthday-time together. Unfortunately, he was having a bad weekend in general. This was even sadder after enjoying my last visit with him as much as I did. Cara and I tried to do the right thing today.

John was at home desperately working on the outside of our house. Having so little spare time for these chores he had no choice but to continue. John may resent some of the time I am allocating to Garry. My husband takes a strong stand on not continuing with the things that we need to do, or missing the fun that might be had, while anguishing through visits with anyone in these types of circumstances. His point is basically: Not to measure devotion in terms of time. He often says, "When it's my turn, I don't want visitors. No one can visit me for more than ten minutes at a time. Don't give up hours, days . . ."

John is definitely concerned about what this situation is taking out of everyone, in particular Mom and Irwin. Most of the time he is fine about my visiting my brother, but there are other things that do require my attention and time. He really does understand, but honestly it is not always easy. John has always loved and respected my brother, so I have no problem with some occasional reluctant support.

This was not a good day at Garry's; even Cara did not seem to brighten him up. We stayed briefly. I did meet Alex's daughter, Ellen. She was the friendly, energetic person he had described. I know Alex will be pleased this encounter finally happened.

On our way out of the home we ran unexpectedly into Cara's friend. He is a terrific sixteen-year-old who is now volunteering at the nursing home on Sundays. What a shame that he never knew Garry before now.

Anne and her boyfriend Dave had planned to come home later to cook us a dinner. We had birthday cake after that with my mom and Irwin stopping by to join us. We ate too much and rushed through to dessert quickly, as it was Sunday evening.

The girls gifted me with a Beatles t-shirt and a copy of *To Kill a Mockingbird*, which I have long wanted to read and has always been one of my favorite movies. Also there was a writing journal to jot down notes when I can't be at the computer. The journal has the "Serenity Prayer," that I have always loved and felt connected to on the cover. Dave made me a DVD he thought I would enjoy. It was all very nice. I remember last year not feeling well from my chemo treatments and canceling out on dinner plans. Wow, what a year! I am very lucky to say the least. Next year . . . less food.

THE SERENITY PRAYER

God, Grant Me the Serenity to

Accept the Things I Cannot Change,

Courage to Change the Things I Can,

And Wisdom to Know the Difference.

This is the part of the Serenity Prayer (by Reinhold Niebuhr) that I have always liked best. After my Dad passed away I found a wrought iron plaque with just those words on it. He had it hanging on his office wall. It is perhaps best known as The Alcoholics' Prayer. It made me happy that the prayer meant something to my Dad, because it always struck a chord with me. Of course, I thought it was a "sign" from him at that time. Maybe this was a reminder-sign?

TREATS AND OTHER SCARY STUFF

It seems to me while preparing for Halloween I become aware that the big holidays are coming up sooner than I thought possible.

Yes, we are buying lots of candies to hand out this weekend. I am committed to not eating any of it early; knowing too well that this holiday consumption is what will determine the accumulation of extra dangerous calories through the rest of the year. The next few weeks tell if the rest of the holidays have even the slightest chance of not doing total damage. As my exercise has been less successful this year, and my diet less controlled, it's going to be tougher. Also the five-year pill, the estrogen blocker, is not helping me feel my best. I can be pretty pessimistic.

Ginny and I got to go for a walk around the track this morning and then she and I went to the store. There I made the candy selections I hoped would offer something for everyone on Halloween. The treats are purchased and kept out of sight from John. He has hidden-goodies radar and usually finds the treasure easily. Hopefully, this candy will be more than enough to see us through the day. Whatever else happens this week—I'm ready to meet all the ghouls with treats on Sunday.

Today, I went a little earlier to see Garry. It was important to me to try and get him outside for some fresh air. It was a beautiful, warm fall day. When I arrived he was waiting in the lunch room. His nurse suggested that I feed him. That was no problem and before we finished Mom and Irwin arrived. Together we went on the patio where Alex soon joined the party. Garry of course, quickly had enough and insisted on getting back upstairs and being put into his bed. He may be slightly jealous of Alex's time with our parents.

Garry's speech is even more difficult to understand and it is turning into a guessing game of sorts. It was disappointing for me to hear he did not go to the music activity at all yesterday and preferred to stay in bed. He is terribly uncomfortable all the time now.

Truthfully, I was glad to make an early exit as there were several errands on my agenda for the afternoon. Weather reports are saying heavy rains tomorrow; I am not planning to go to Garry's again until Wednesday. I tried to emphasize that I am uncomfortable about coming out to see him in bad weather. Rain would not necessarily stop me from traveling. However, I was hoping to make the point for Mom to take the cue also. He must try and understand that Mom and Irwin should not have to travel on bad days. He has to expect that every now and then, we may not be able to come by. Especially as the winter weather becomes a factor.

Most residents don't have the constant daily company Garry has come to expect. He is much younger than other residents, leaving him more socially connected. As I say these things, I am also thinking about whether Garry will be with us much longer. It is amazing that he has lasted in this condition. Certainly *I* don't have a clue what to expect. Recently I read that ALS is usually a two—five-year disease. We are guessing that it has been about two years since certain symptoms started to appear.

This morning there was more on my mind than immediately deciding what time to leave to see my brother. An overdose of caffeine yesterday and dozens of thoughts about things spiraling out of my control prevented me from falling off to sleep and getting some desperately needed "Zzzzzzs."

I also needed to get to some long-neglected jobs. My medical papers were in desperate need of updating. I know it won't be long before certain information will need to be gathered. I spent over three hours just sifting through the pile. It is not finished. Organization is always difficult for me and I have been trying to work out a better system for the last year-and-a-half. Right now, I feel like I'm losing this battle.

It seems funny when I started this journal to document my experiences with breast cancer; I imagined that the project would take me through the second surgery and that recovery. I now see how much longer this "road" is than I had anticipated. In addition my appreciation for how much I am enjoying writing is much greater than I could have ever expected. I have come to understand how impactful my brother's crisis is on our family. It is clear to me that my issues now pale greatly in comparison.

This project has become more about a period of time when our family and friends have had to deal with some of the most difficult challenges we have ever had. When I think about some of the other problems that have come up during this same time, it has been an unusually stressful period. Writing has been very helpful. It really reinforces many important feelings and facts that I don't want to forget; it also helps me keep a strong sense of perspective about our lives.

Regrettably, my sister and I appear to have lost the extremely close connection we were enjoying. I feel sad about that—I know better than to try and insert myself when she is redirected. It may be that she is not coping with Garry's situation very well. I feel guilty she may have ended up resenting the time and energy my situation cost her. It is unlikely, but you don't know what someone else is thinking.

John stayed home on Wednesday. To my surprise, he had a doctor's appointment for an annual checkup. Afterward he decided it was too late to head to the office and decided he could be more productive at home.

It turned out to be a gorgeous autumn afternoon and we worked together outside. It was such a great day that even *I* did not mind the yard work. John loved being able to have at least one beautiful fall day to enjoy. His job has been forcing him to work lots of overtime recently. He loves to be outside and moving about as much as possible when he is not on the job.

Given the size of this cleanup job he was particularly happy to have my help. After a while my arms and shoulders were definitely feeling the strain of the extra exertion. Later in the evening I felt the pain of overdoing the raking. Maybe I'm still healing; hopefully this will get better with time. It seems that nerve damage from the mastectomy and sentinel lymph node removal may cause some of these issues. The fingers on my right hand were actually numb all night long.

I have started to notice that sleeping on my side is getting a little easier and less painful. I can spend some time asleep before I have to readjust my position. Hey, it is some improvement at least.

This morning Laura came and picked me up to go visit Garry. First, we had a late breakfast together at a diner on the way to the nursing home. Laura insisted on treating me for my birthday. We both enjoy this tradition and rigidly stick to it. She is the best. She brought along a huge smiley-face balloon to place in Garry's bedroom window.

My brother was glad to see Laura. Garry appeared weaker and more tired than ever. This was my fourth visit this week and I think he is declining each time. He is following the conversations and responding sparingly to direct questions. He spends most of the day in bed and is less engaged in generally. It seemed to both Laura and I that his breathing was more labored today. Mom stayed with us. Irwin sat with his buddy Alex in the lounge area listening to some of the great music of long ago. They are both hard of hearing and take turns falling asleep.

Mom gave my brother ice cream, which she has started to allow him to have again. It is her bargaining tool. He has to be nicer to the staff, and then she will reward him in the afternoon with this little indulgence. She also gave him some juice. We were especially glad to see to him drinking some fluid as he constantly perspires heavily. It is always a welcome visit with Laura, but today it felt sadder than our past visits.

Earlier in the week I spoke with the hospice-aide who told me she thought Garry was "winding down." At the same time she suggested that we might want to spend a little less time with him, so that he might become better bonded to the home. She seemed to think if this happened he might be more comfortable about being here. This gal is very sincere and I am sure she excels at her work. Her vagueness confused me and perhaps I may not have been bold enough to ask the "right" questions of her. In addition, her accent and gentle demeanor makes communication a little unclear at times.

Garry does not want to be there and does not like most of the staff at all. He is miserable and frankly, I do not think the "comfort-bonding thing" is ever going to happen. It is a horrible problem as the staff, I believe, does not fully understand how mentally intelligent, alert, and sensitive he is.

I am reminded of my Dad when was bed-ridden right before he died. He asked me for help in turning slightly as he was in severe pain. He looked at me as he ground his teeth and said, "There is really no dignity in dying." Of course, my father understood and accepted his situation better than my brother is able to do. What I assumed my dad was referring to was at the very end, when he needed help and was in constant pain. Maybe he meant the whole damn thing! He had been a realistic and undemanding patient.

Obviously, I am thinking more than usual about my Dad lately. He was only fifty-eight when he died. Like Garry I believe he accomplished so much in a short life. Given their individual talents and opportunities, they were more successful than most people are. Certainly I am not considering those successes in monetary ways; they were both really special, dedicated human beings. Wow, being reflective takes a lot out of me—it is definitely time to get some needed sleep.

Saturday Cara and I made a short trip to see Garry. My suspicion is that he was doing especially poorly this past week. We felt the need to spend some time with him and I hoped Cara might be a welcome guest. He was still lethargic and did not perk up much at all. Mom, Cara and I basically talked and he either stared at the TV, or closed his eyes and just listened. The oxygen was hooked up to him today, and it appeared that his breathing was slightly easier than yesterday. I told him that tomorrow is Halloween and he should not expect to see me. This did not seem to create any problem for him. We left feeling a bit empty about the visit.

Next, I dropped Cara off to meet some friends. It is Cabbage Night (Mischief Night) tonight. I have never let my children out for this accepted form of trashing others property and such. It is a pet peeve of mine. However, I did let her meet her friends in the afternoon knowing that they were likely to all spend the rest of the evening together. Cara is stressing about all the typical teenage drama lately, and I thought she needed some time with her buddies.

Cara called saying that she was going to "just hang out" at her friend's house and that they had no plans of carousing. I told her that their plan was fine. She came home via a ride from her first close friend to become a licensed driver just this week. Now that is scary! My big worry is about Anne and Keith finding out that Cara was out this evening. Surely, there will be some choice backlash on this one. Oy!

Halloween was oddly quiet. The past several years we have found less and less trick or treaters coming to our area. We live in a nice area, but not the wealthiest one of our town. Supposedly, the wealthier areas are drawing a larger crowd. With the effects of the economy I'm not sure you can tell which homes are faring the best.

Cara and her friends were out a very short time. They did not seem to be into the whole running-around thing.

Anne and Dave went to the Zombie Parade on the beach at Asbury Park on Saturday. They were amazed to see how many people participated dressed as zombies and ghost brides. The spirited group of all ages did a *"Thriller"* dance that made the trip well worthwhile.

Halloween day they came home to get some key pointers on using the subway system from John. Then they went to another parade in the city and called us later to say that all worked out great. Anne's sense of adventure definitely does not come from us. I do think it is admirable for the most part. Of course, I was nervous about the plan until it was all over.

Keith remained at school to attend several parties there.

Wow! It is November already! Yikes, we are talking about the big holidays, which are fast approaching. This makes me think of all that I have to do. I want to just go back to bed. But, I had to get some things done. It was a day of food shopping, errands, and changing summer to winter clothes at long last. It was good to have the entire day being more productive.

It may be awful of me, but I'm starting to feel that the time I spend with Garry is not bringing him any real comfort. I am sure it helps my Mom, but it is getting more difficult for me. It is easier for us all when I bring company.

We have a meeting about Garry at the nursing home tomorrow. On Wednesday I will pick Mom up to go over to Garry as Irwin has a doctor's appointment that he has to go to. With the knowledge of spending part of the next two days with my brother I felt confident that I could do some of my own tasks today.

Tuesday's "care meeting" at the nursing home went as we might have wanted and expected. The report was: Garry is relatively stable although his overall condition is declining. The pain patch he is now wearing seems to be keeping him more comfortable. The staff wants us to offer Garry very small amounts of soda and an ice cream each day as "comfort." This made me suspicious that it is even nearer to the end. They made it clear that we must be careful because of his choking problems.

We talked vaguely about how much time Garry has left. No one can be sure. The staff told us they know "Garry is a very special person." It meant a lot to my Mom to hear this. Apparently, his negative nature and his new-found penchant for cursing at people is not something that they take personally. We tried to show our appreciation for their efforts. I felt that they were trying hard to be sensitive to our needs, too.

Our social worker told us about a conversation he had with an unnamed resident. The man was not happy and the social worker asked, "What is it that you want?" To which he got this reply, "I want *that.*" The older man was pointing at my mother and Irwin. They had been listening, holding hands, and dancing to the music in the social hall that afternoon. Obviously this was shared to offer something meaningful to us today.

My folks have made the best of these months in the nursing home making many friends and acquaintances; they participate and are cheerful whenever possible. Irwin said, "It is the most fun we could have while being miserable; believe it or not." He always added, "Ya have to find something to laugh about or you'll go crazy!"

I texted my sister to let her know there was a meeting and asked her to give me a call to bring her up to speed. She called me back minutes later to find out what was going on. Quickly the call went in the wrong direction and she was impatient and curt. Vicki is an expert on everything and one must remember that fact in most conversations. She was particularly unhappy about the decision to allow Garry to drink soda and concerned about his frequent choking. She said she was also upset about us feeding him ice cream while on oxygen. This puzzled me. It is definitely the case that while he is having a problem, he should not be fed. My sister was in an antagonistic state.

After a number of her nasty remarks, I told her that I did not want to continue the discussion. She shot back with an abrupt and angry response about how busy she was and did not have time to talk . . . I hung up. This is something I don't do to her, ever. She is the most incredibly generous person in some ways and she is also terribly selfish in others. Her extremes often exasperate me, but usually I deal with them silently.

Most recently, she is the person who got me through every appointment and procedure for the entire first year of my breast cancer. It would have been so much more difficult for me if she had not been there. It was wonderful that the situation allowed us to feel amazingly close to one another again. I will *always* treasure her support.

Now though, I am annoyed with her. Of course, I realize how rude I was to her on the phone and honestly, it makes me feel terrible. However, I'm not going to beat myself up about this one. Vicki is going to have to understand she is not last word on everything. This kind of tension and disagreement may be common among people trying to get through similar circumstances. Things are so stressful and getting worse!

Mom expected me to take her to see Garry today. John and I decided that my first stop would have to be to the bank. We have been waiting on a loan authorization for about six weeks or so. A couple of weeks ago we were told our paperwork was lost. With several attempts by phone John tried to find out where we stood. If we do not sign and return our papers in less than one week we will lose a chunk of money, which we cannot afford to do. Ah, more problems.

There is the long list of household problems that keep growing and now this is "the last straw." My mission was to go to both banks and figure out how to expedite this paperwork. After over two hours I managed to explain our situation. We finally found that the banks were not agreeing on a particular form and we needed to straighten this glitch out.

It seems to me that nothing gets taken care of without fighting your way through whatever needs to be done. It is shocking how many people do not know how to do their job. Funny, how fast both these banks had taken our money to get the "ball rolling."

I know this should be our worst problem, but it is very disturbing piled on top of everything else that we are dealing with. Also, while I am venting: How the heck do people get these things taken care of when both spouses have full-time jobs? When I think how much time I spend on medical issues, household repair problems, additional errands, and more—it is amazing. No wonder we are all "losing it!" Could John have ever given the time to address this problem? Certainly not and actually do the job he gets paid to do at the same time. Am I trying to justify my present situation? This is enough journaling for today.

HOLDING MY BREATH

Mom and I went to visit Garry as planned after my business with the banks was taken care of. He seemed a little better this afternoon. The new pain patch makes him much more comfortable. He was more present and appeared slightly more content. He managed to smile several times and actually broke out in some quiet laughing twice. That helps me feel that these visits are still important and gratifying.

I told mom and Garry lots of stories about the times the kids got in trouble through the years. I am still hoping their lessons were learned. But, today I appreciated the old stories for our conversation and entertainment.

My friend Marian sent me a gift of food. I called her immediately to thank her. We spoke briefly as she was busy. Marian wanted me to know she thinks of me often, despite the fact that we don't get the chance to see one another. I understand her busy life and likewise she appreciates my current obligations.

Even when so many things are going poorly there are nice things happening, too. Though it took a while, that idea finally slipped back in to my consciousness.

I'm anxiety ridden from the bank dilemma. John has declared that these are the type of problems he deals with as a daily routine and he said, "I'm not going to worry about the outcome." He is trying to remain impervious to allowing this kind of problem getting to him and feels that if it goes wrong we will figure a way through that, too. I am exhausted and mistrusting.

I waited until 10:00 this morning and started to make phone calls to follow up on what was going on. In the midst of the whole process I connected with a supervisor who really was most helpful at our original bank. She kept on top of things for two days. She saw to expediting the file until it concluded in our being approved and sent it back to the other bank. Ah, communication is a wonderful thing!

Ginny called me early and I shared the bank dilemma with her. She and I have a running joke going on about how unprofessional and incompetent people are at their jobs. It is not that we think we are perfect or so smart. We just are amazed at how much time and involvement is required to make things work the way they are supposed to.

Then, Colette called for the first time in weeks. We have been trading text messages. She and I had a lengthy conversation about how her mom and my brother are doing. Both are not expected to be with us for much longer. We are thinking about the upcoming holidays and how difficult they will be for everyone.

Colette sincerely tries to offer the encouragement and wisdom she has gained from her own journey and experience. We decided to get together next week and visit Garry. She desperately wants my mother to go to see her mom and I feel awful about that. Mom will never agree to the trip which requires a total of approximately four hours of driving. Normally yes, she would do this for her neighbor and friend of over fifty years. But, with daily visits to Garry, I know this will become a denied request.

There is a part of me that understands both of their feelings on this subject. My friend is hurt that many people have not kept in touch with her mother. My mom has continued to correspond by mail. It is understandable that Colette would like to bring her mom as much comfort as possible. My mother knows full well how important visitors have been for Garry.

As Garry's communication becomes more limited it obviously makes visitors less at ease. Everyone does their best, and we are grateful that many people continue to stop by. Colette seemed happy to know I would accompany her for a second visit to see her mom. It is the least I can do for them both.

Cara and I were out doing errands and eventually were going by my brother for a short visit. The day quickly slipped away. It was too late for Cara who had plans for this part of the day and I went by myself.

This visit was surprisingly good with my brother. Mom, Garry and I sat and talked for a while. He is more comfortable with the effective new pain patches. He asked questions when he was not sure of something said and made comments; what a difference this was. He was very funny as Irwin came in and we started to talk about who would win the big 50-50 raffle the nursing home is running this Sunday. Garry kept insisting that he wants John to win because he really needs to buy a new car. Well, guess what? John has not bought one raffle ticket. *"Ya' gotta be in it, to win it!"* We had a few chuckles over the possibilities.

A staffer came into Garry's room for the first time and she was amazed at how cheerful the room is. She commented on all the balloons, cards and pictures. She said, "Garry no wonder you want to stay in your room, it's so cheerful!" Garry replied, "Now, you know why I like to be in here." She reminded him that she still would like him to come out and join in some activities.

Then she commented on how great his family and friends have been to come by so often and he replied, "Not all. I have one friend who hasn't been so good." He continued by saying, "I went to see her mom all the time when she was sick, too." This was the biggest conversation he has had in a while. It was not easy to understand him and we made a collective effort to do this.

It broke my heart to hear this friend was on his mind. He had made me phone her and leave messages about where he was, but she never responded. We told him that some people cannot cope well seeing their loved ones sick and don't know what to do. We told him to feel good knowing that he had been a good friend. It makes me wonder what else he is thinking about in his forced silence. Generally, it was a rewarding visit.

By the late afternoon I received a number of calls regarding the loan. All systems appear to be "go." Monday morning I need to confirm this and bring the signed papers to the bank. Then we will close by early December. It was an exhausting week.

Anne was expected for a rare dinner with John and me. Cara was out with her "posse," which is how she often refers to her group of friends. So, it is not quite a full boat tonight, but that was OK.

We were in the middle of dinner with Anne on Friday night when Keith came in at the tail end. We talked about all sorts of things. Keith informed us that a second operation is needed to fix an ACL tear. The doctor could not evaluate the ACL properly before due to the great amount of swelling caused by the original injury. Oh, I wasn't happy about that. It does seem that this is a smaller procedure than the last one.

Saturday John needed help on his outdoor work and Keith, Cara and I joined the effort. Keith lent John a hand on a huge job that John is doing around the siding of our house. Cara and I worked on blowing the leaves out of the garden and raking them up. Gardening is not my favorite activity, but it was good to know we were helping out in some way.

Sunday we all went to see Garry for a short visit. Of course, it went longer than I had thought it would. He was pleased to see everyone and appeared more sociable and calm. John and Keith were relieved to see this slight improvement as they engaged my brother in conversation. Mom and I did a bit of shopping at the craft-show fundraiser at the home.

There were great hopes, on all our parts, that we would share the raffle win by the end of the day. I finally agreed to double my chances and vice versa with Irwin's plan of pooling the tickets.

By the time we got back home and ate a late lunch together we decided that more outdoor work was not going to take place today. Perhaps it was that the clocks were set back today and we all felt it was later. Keith and I ran out to the pharmacy for our annual flu shots. It made me feel better knowing he got this done. Anyway, the weekend was good and Keith took off and went back to school by early evening. It would seem that neither Irwin, nor I won the raffle. Gee, what a surprise!

My agenda today is to go to the bank with our signed papers, which will be delivered on time. This was the result of some collective energy, enormous hassle, and juggling on our and the bank's part.

Laura came at noon to visit my brother. Mom and Irwin will not be there for the day. They are needed to remain at home while they have some repair work completed. This is literally the second day in about five months that they have not been with Garry. Hopefully, knowing Laura and I are spending the afternoon with him provides my mom with some peace of mind.

Later, Cara will need a ride back to school where her appointment for her audition for this year's play will be at 6:30. She has a cold which might affect how this goes. Cara will do well no matter what. It is clear that she is fairly nervous. This is the "normal" stuff that happens each year.

Anne just called sounding quite sick; she will go to the doctor in a little while. It is likely that I will postpone my doctor's appointment on Wednesday because she should not sit in the oncology waiting room. We will know more after her appointment. While I am waiting and "holding my breath," I'm trying not to stress!

The afternoon with Garry and Laura went fine. We found him to be very agreeable today. His new chair pad finally arrived and it seemed to make him more comfortable. It was the first day in a long time he was able to stay up in his special hospital chair after lunch. We pleased him with a second smuggled-in portion of rice pudding. He was definitely more content after that. He even agreed to go to the music activity for the first time in three weeks.

If he was unhappy that Mom and Irwin were not there too, we did not know it. Later though, he was disappointed to learn that their job at home was not completed and they were not expecting to come by.

After a little time Garry said he had enough music and wanted to return to his room again. We made sure to have him put back into his bed. He was tired and still using the oxygen. It always seems to make him more secure to be back in bed with the TV on fairly loudly while he waits for his dinner in his room. He dislikes the common food area and is uncomfortable listening to people complaining about wanting to go back to their rooms. Once he is back in bed he feels safer. His favorite TV station is always left on for him. We placed a note on the top of the TV his first day here, requesting this particular station, in case it is changed or accidentally turned off.

My mother called a couple of times throughout the day and it was obvious that she was filled with angst. We made sure he was as comfortable as possible and then said our goodbyes. It was an above average visit.

Laura brought me some amazing homemade pumpkin cheesecake. Wow! She is getting to be a very bad influence!

Anne was put on an antibiotic for a sinus infection. She cannot go to work for a couple of days. As Colette had offered to help me out with a ride to the city if ever I got in a jam, I decided to call her. I knew it was an imposition. My appointment could be postponed; however, with Anne's court date, the bank closing, and the holidays this might get tricky. Colette was agreeable and said, "It will give us a good opportunity to chat." Things really do have a way of working out most of the time. My friends are awesome!

After some discussion at home, John and I decided to call Tom and Barbara. Plans for Thanksgiving were not settled and it needed to be figured out. She and I decided the holiday would be at our house this year. It was best so that my mother and Irwin could join us after whatever time they spend with Garry.

As of now, I have not spoken to my sister in two weeks. This is hard for me, I am wearing thin on many levels, and the last thing I need is my sister acting so unreasonably. In fact I *wanted* to step into Garry's issues, so that she would feel comfortable knowing that I was helping Mom when she cannot. It was a perfect way to pay Vicki back for all she had done for me.

However, I draw the line at her yelling at me! Guess I can definitely hold my breath on her getting in touch with me. I am not upset with her or the reasons behind her behavior. We are all stressed!

Knowing that my doctor's appointment will keep me from stopping over to see Garry on Wednesday, I did go by for a very quick visit today. Mom and Irwin and Alex were all in the lounge talking and listening to music. Garry was still in the lunch room. Mom eventually brought him to sit with us for a little while. He seemed much more tired and weaker today.

I have seen him many days when he appeared to be getting worse; then, another day he seems better again. I don't want to jump to any conclusions. He had some visitors after Laura and I left yesterday. Perhaps, all the company wore him out. There was an expression in his eyes that unnerved me. I felt as though he wanted to say something, but he couldn't. This short visit left me feeling unsettled as I walked to my car.

Cara came home with the news that she has call-backs for several parts in this year's play. It was hard to figure out whether "several" was good or not. The next auditions are on Monday after school.

I am feeling like I should not have asked Colette to help me out tomorrow. Also I dread the talk I must have with the Oncologist about my medication. It is apparent to me that the side effects are unacceptable and continuing is questionable in my mind. The doctor will have to tell me what the next option could be regarding this aspect of the treatment.

November 10, Colette drove me into New York. She is an aggressive driver and the city did not intimidate her one bit. We were early and so the wait was longer. We were busy talking until I was called in to see my oncologist. I told my doctor and her "fellow" doctor about my discomfort with the estrogen blocker medication. My complaints were muscle and joint pain, headaches and sleeplessness.

Unfortunately, the muscle and joint pains could be from issues that I had prior to my diagnosis of breast cancer. Sleep has been a problem since surgery but this is different. This is unrelated to pain or waking from discomfort. It is just like a caffeine-overdose-exhaustion with no chance of getting a wink.

In addition, I told her that I am very stressed out with personal problems and I wasn't sure of *anything*. My doctor reminded me that she had initially told me, "The pill is more important than the chemotherapy, in your case. It reduces the risks almost fifty percent against any future new breast cancer." She said the chemo was my choice; this she felt more strongly about. She advised me to stop taking the medication for four weeks. After one week off the medicine I should start to see a difference if my symptoms are from that.

If there is indication of a problem with this drug, another medication will be prescribed for me. If not, then I will likely continue with this one. I must go back in one month to have bloodwork, and we will decide what should be done. As always, I felt very confident that this doctor was listening to me.

After my appointment Colette and I stopped in the restaurant across the street from the doctor's offices to have a late lunch. By the time we got home it was already late afternoon. We talked till we had to say goodbye, but we could have easily continued. Next week we will visit her Mom on Wednesday and have more time. This trip today was such a big help. It is one thing to do a favor; it is another to really make someone feel like they are not asking much of you.

When I got home I decided I would bite the bullet and send my sister a text. The text I sent Vicki only said, "We plan to have Thanksgiving and we would like you three to come." It did not include any mention of the last phone call. My hope is that she will realize this is a terrible time for such nonsense. I will hold my breath on this one for sure!

I woke up to two text messages. One was from Laura, who asked how Cara made out on her audition. That was sweet of her; I will keep my friend posted on how the play is going.

The second was a simple message back from Vicki. It said that they are having the holiday with Jennifer in the city. She did say, "Thanks, hope all is well." We are most likely on the same page. That's as good as you get. I feel better about this, as the last thing we all need is more family stress.

GATHERING UP STEAM

My day was filled with errands. Plans to visit Garry were interrupted as I was easily sidetracked by some shopping along the way. After figuring out how to use my new navigation device last night we decided that I should purchase a special mounting accessory and carrying case.

After I completed that mission, I made an additional stop to pick up some chocolates to bring when I see Etta next week. I managed to go to a store that also had lots of Christmas items and I found the cutest snowman holding a big heart. I intend to include him with what I give to Colette's mom. I love snowmen that are filled with personality. They are nice through the long winter months.

It was likely that Cara would stay after school and I would need to go pick her up. Looking at the time, I knew I could make one more shopping stop. I found several items for Anne that will be put away for her as part of her Christmas presents. Wow, I never start this early. The snowman must have made me do it!

The real work of my day did not get done. The bills and other tasks will have to wait. Tomorrow, no matter what, I'm heading out to see Garry.

It was Friday and I had not seen my brother since Tuesday. Mom and Irwin were in the lobby just waiting for Garry to finish his lunch. They looked so worn out which caused me some extra concern. They came with me to get coffee in the café and we sat and waited until we thought it was time to head upstairs. We were all especially tired today.

For my own part, I had only two hours of sleep; it had been one of those nights where I felt exhausted and I lay concentrating on problem after problem. At one point I thought to get up and take a pill, but resisted making the noise of getting to them. I'm still reluctant about taking them. By about 2:00 in the morning a headache forced me to get up to take something for that. Seated on the den couch, I continued to do all the things in my head which I have been procrastinating about actually doing.

The next day I got to Garry just as he had been put back in bed. He was screaming and yelling as the aide was attending to him. He was in pain and angry about being handled. Even with his room door closed, it was the worst I have heard him and that says a lot. This was torturous for Mom, Irwin and I as we waited to see him.

By the time we saw him, he was choking continuously. Garry panics and though we all try to remain calm, it is often quite scary to witness. The combination of the heavy amount of fluid he is producing in his throat and the deteriorating muscles creates a very serious condition. Even in the midst of a bad time he will insist on a drink, a mouthful of soup, or ice cream. It is an extremely disconcerting experience. Really awful!

Garry was particularly demanding and I tried to remain firm with him. I tried explaining that we couldn't give him anything while he is choking, no matter what he said. Mom was shot and I think my presence was making her more nervous. By 2:30 I made my goodbyes saying I had to leave to do some more errands. Maybe it was unfair on my part, but today it was all too much for me.

When I got back home I received a telephone call. It was Carol and Peter, wanting to know how Garry was. My cousin has been incredibly generous and supportive toward the organization that owns and operates the group home in which my brother had lived. Our family is indebted to him for this.

Carol also wanted me to know that she will be away in January when she had wanted to take Cara to see her alma mater. She hoped I would take my daughter there anyway. This was not a problem and I assured her we would make the trip.

By the way, today's mail brought lots of the usual and one surprise. Cara got into the National Honor Society. It was wonderful to share this news with my cousins and they were excited for her.

I can imagine Keith's reaction when he hears this news as he hates those bumper stickers "I am the Proud Parent of an Honor Student." Keith will really be happy for his sister; they love to give one another a hard time and still be supportive.

—ᴡᴡ—

Well, I am feeling so successful! My new GPS and I are now friends. This could be the beginning of a "beautiful friendship." It was simpler to use than I anticipated because I am fearful of all new gadgets. It needed a destination to be tried out; I set it to take me to Garry's. Tonight I need to pick Cara and a few other people up from a high school I have never been to before. It forces me to drive to a town that I am completely unfamiliar with. This was the perfect day to have my new and valuable tool.

The kids are all a part of the play critic's group that Cara has joined this year. They watch different school productions, and critique them in a written review format. At the end of the season, they will nominate and vote for different categories at a Tony Awards-like ceremony. Viewing the productions will provide good exposure to what other schools are doing. It should be a great experience on many levels requiring time, energy, cooperation and objectivity.

Tonight is Cara's first show to critique. I am fully ready with my new gadget to pick them up later tonight. I think it will be invaluable for me with my poor sense of direction. This was the first test. Untechno-Girl is off!

The destination of Garry's home worked well. It allowed me to alter my route and listen to the prompts to be sure it was all working well. My arrival was on a gorgeous, mild autumn day. It was a nice stroll from my car to the main entrance. When I got to his room my brother was in bed. Mom and Irwin went to visit Alex for a few minutes. Garry appeared calm but somber. He said he was having a bad day. It was apparent he was not happy Mom and Irwin were out of sight; it seemed likely that they needed to distance themselves from him.

Garry would barely look at me, but he managed to ask about the children and I gave him the usual run-down. When my folks came back they looked totally stressed out. We talked for about another twenty minutes or more, and then we all said goodbye. Garry was annoyed. Mom said they were very tired and needed to get going. They shopped in the morning for more pajama bottoms for Garry, and then came to see him earlier today. They were ready to go home. I instinctively felt my leaving was best and wanted to walk them out to their car.

It had been at least two unusually difficult days with Garry. Leaving when he is not in the midst of any problems with either breathing or choking is much easier. I completely understood. Their strain was obvious.

That night Cara called for us to pick her group up from the show. Confidently, I went to the car to enter our new destination. This time I could not enter the address. My meltdown began and by the time John got into the car I was convinced that I was a complete jackass.

Luckily, Cara had printed out directions from the Internet just in case we needed them. We started out following those directions. After some trial and error John figured out how to enter the information correctly. We were back in business. We arrived before they finished. I was glad that John came with me as this trip would have been problematic. Anyway, my GPS will be a huge help.

Cara and her friends were wound up and talked about the play most of the way home. They each have to submit a review by tomorrow. The mentors will pick the reviews that will be published in that school's newspaper.

Sunday, Mary called and we caught up with each other. After dealing with her medical issues for well over a year, she was finally feeling markedly better. We saw each other a couple of weeks ago at Bob's Mom's funeral, but we hadn't spoken much since. She and I often speak to each other on Sundays, except lately this has been almost impossible.

John and Bob went out to hit some golf balls. I was surprised that John agreed to take time off from the work around the outside of the house. The weather was ideal and most likely there won't be many more quite this mild. He needed the break and really deserved one. John would stop by to visit Garry afterward, as he would be very close to the nursing home.

I went to see Garry too because it was unlikely that I would make it to see him for a few days. Also, I was concerned that John would never understand anything Garry said, making it harder on them both. Mom and Irwin were leaving the complex, and Vicki and Jen had left an hour before that. When I arrived Garry was sleeping. He woke up the minute I entered but was very tired. He did not perk up with me. We sat together and watched TV until John came in.

John automatically rubbed Garry's feet and ankles, which brought an instant and long-lasting smile to my brother's face. It shocked me that he could even do this much. Our visit was short. My brother was barely able to engage in any dialog. He may have been worn out from all the visitors this afternoon.

It felt like Garry was starting to disappear and that left me feeling sad. John and I never spoke about how depleted he seemed today. I was thankful John was able to do something to make my brother comfortable and happier for a few minutes.

Monday I waited for the dishwasher repairman. I hoped that it needed only a simple switch or fuse. It seemed fortunate to have this done before the holiday next week. The man came and quickly informed me that I was looking at a large and foolishly wasteful repair. My next step was to spend the rest of the afternoon purchasing a replacement. Doesn't that put the "thanks" in Thanksgiving?

Tuesday was our closing on the new mortgage. John had taken the day off. Since it was nasty and rainy out we knew we would work on a few other problems besides the outdoor projects. We were on a roll, needing a new dishwasher, mortgage, shower door and vacuum. John's shower repair had gone badly (twice) and there was no way another attempt would be made. After the ridiculous expenses of the last couple of days, it seemed like buying a new vacuum was just a perfect way to end the day. Well, the dishes and floors should be in better shape for the holiday.

The toughest part of the week's trials was finding the time for visiting my brother. Wednesday, November 17, I went to see Colette's Mom as planned. She appeared weaker, more tired, and less sociable than she was at the end of June. She was on oxygen, and after lunch she needed to go back into her bed and take a short nap.

I gifted Etta with the chocolates and the snowman, which she liked. Colette cut and curled her mom's hair and helped her write a card. She was great at assisting her mom. Colette frequently adjusted her oxygen wires and the general positioning of her mother. It was nice to see how lovingly she attended to all of this. I felt badly as I thought this might be my last visit with her mom. But, we never know what will be, do we? I'm glad I accompanied my friend. Neither of us has had an easy time of things for a while, and it is comforting to discuss our mutual concerns.

Thursday we are expecting the new dishwasher. An early delivery will mean I can still make a visit to Garry. The man is coming Friday to measure the shower area for the new doors in the afternoon. Yikes this is making me crazy, as I want my time to do what is most important to me and all these extra issues are getting in the way.

The next two nights I will be at school at a monthly meeting and at a fundraiser I felt obligated to attend. Cara will be out with the critics' group both those nights, and has offered me to pick up at the end of tomorrow's show and discussion. I don't mind, because I would rather not miss the fundraiser the next evening. What a hectic week!

My Mom has called every day with reports of Garry saying less and less. He is sleeping much more of the time now. Her frustration is great, but she is understanding and seems OK with my absence. She never complains, yet her voice sounds stressed and tired.

My dishwasher never came as they called to say that the one on their truck was damaged and they needed to reschedule for Saturday. Now, I'm able to see Garry. First, I will stop and pick up some new balloons for his room. Usually he seems pleased by this cheery touch. I have been changing the balloons about every seven to ten days.

Garry actually was better today than I had expected. My suspicion is that at his weight, he is strongly affected by the pain medication he is on. As it wears off he is more engaged and less sleepy.

I refreshed his balloons while he was still out of his room. Laura's big smiley-faced balloon deflated drastically over the past week. He accepted its removal, but wanted me to know he noticed. He spoke sparingly and smiled at various comments we made. When I told him that Cara's review was one of two selected for the school newspaper he confidently remarked, "I knew they would pick hers."

I rubbed my brother's feet as we sat together. The hope was to bring him some pleasure. Maybe John gives a better foot massage, because Garry did not have the same smile on his face. He was quite alert and it was a relief to me that I found him this way. Mom had really worried me describing him constantly sleeping and not speaking much for days now. While Garry definitely wants our company he may also be bored with Mom, Irwin and I. Now that is pretty hard to believe, right?

This visit was a few hours long and then I was off to do some errands. When I left Mom was with Garry and Irwin was with Alex. Irwin was sound asleep while his pal was enjoying this month's birthday celebration program. We found out that Alex will be turning only eighty-nine and not ninety as we originally thought on November 29, which makes him younger than Irwin by three months. This fact has not changed their friendship in any measurable way.

The next few days brought un-newsworthy and regular events. The high school's annual music fundraiser was very enjoyable. We asked our friends Maryann and Tony to join us. Anne and Cara went to see the new Harry Potter movie together as is their tradition. Saturday our new dishwasher came. Wow, I was happy to see that after an entire week of hand washing!

Today both Anne and Cara wanted to visit Garry with me. Cara and I went on our own so she could practice driving first. She was rusty and I was not as patient as I should have been.

We spent a short time with Garry before Anne and Dave stopped in. Mom and Irwin had been there for a while already. Garry was quiet, but fairly comfortable. He asked about Laura coming this week and I told him I thought she would likely come next week. I think he was hoping to have more pudding. Cara and I left first, as I needed to start my holiday food shopping. We made that our next stop. I have a long list of things to do before Thursday. Finding time to visit will be tough but I will do my best.

Mom did not want Garry to know that I was hosting the holiday. She thinks he will be very upset about missing the day. This makes my absence for the next few days more mysterious. Oh, how I wish he were coming over like so many other Thanksgivings. He was always anxious to load up on my mashed potatoes!

Back in the Saddle Again

Thanksgiving was nice and very manageable as we were a small group. We expected Rita and our nephews, Dan and Rob, Tom and Barbara and my Mom and Irwin. Mom, Irwin, Vicki, Paul and Jen saw Garry earlier in the afternoon. After that Mom and Irwin came to our home for the holiday dinner. Though we were all saddened about Garry's absence, it still turned out well.

My sisters-in-law brought lots of food contributions helping me out tremendously. Most of all, Anne had taken the day before off from work to help out here. We worked together all day. We cooked, straightened up and set up as much as possible. Cara helped, but Anne and I did the bulk of the preparations. We were ready.

The holiday was easier for me as a result of everyone's efforts. Anne unfortunately, was exhausted! The children, who range from sixteen to twenty-five, were great company and kept things very upbeat. Our niece Mary Kate was missing as she was attending a semester in London—lucky girl! Mom and Irwin were tired, but able to appreciate the opportunity to be with everyone. Hosting the holiday was a sign that my life was returning to "normal." The celebration worked out for everybody. My sister texted me later on to say they were not coming by. That was fine as they often chose to be absent on Thanksgiving.

Deservedly, Anne was proud of all her contributions to the day. Sorry to say, she was beyond pooped from being such a great help and probably enjoyed herself less than she might have. Next time, I will make her go easier.

Keith was home for the long weekend. We were glad to have him home as he had not been here much this semester. Recovery, less driving, and a heavy school-work load made him a scarce visitor. He seemed quite good despite still needing physical therapy for his leg.

Before leaving to head back to school, Keith brought the Christmas tree down from the attic, and set it up in the living room window as we have done for years. We were determined to keep everything as normal as possible. This year I added more lights to the tree and it was gorgeous! We all felt in better spirits almost immediately.

Anne's court date came in the beginning of December. It was a difficult experience for her. She was an emotional wreck that day; her lawyer asked the judge to postpone the case to a private hearing date. The judge agreed, which meant this case would be closed to the general public. The court had not hired the requested interpreter for the defendant—most likely the process would have been delayed anyway.

We were not given a new date and left feeling this problem remained unresolved. The prosecutor told Anne next time he plans to meet her before the court appearance and will prepare her. He explained, "If you can't tell your story there is no case." His advice was, "Stop acting like a victim and get angry and be more in control."

My friends Laura and Colette continued to visit Garry with me. Their visits were important to him and they really helped brighten Mom and Irwin's day. Laura remarked about noticing the decline in my brother's condition and said, "These visits mean so much to me also. I love Garry—he has been wonderful to me for years and I feel like he is a part of my family. These times have given me a chance to know your mom and Irwin better; it forced us all to spend more time together and I love that." I know how deeply she feels, and there are no words to say how much this has meant to me.

Colette's visits also comfort my mom as they have known each other for a long time. Mom has gained a greater affection for our former neighbor and friend during these times. I told my friend that I was concerned Garry might not be with us in the New Year; she thought me wrong. Colette fussed gently over my brother trying to make him as comfortable as possible. All the experience she has with her mother has made her a considerate and caring visitor.

John's Aunt Betty has sent Garry cards throughout his crisis. In addition, she occasionally calls mom to speak to her directly. We are all so fond of her. She is amazing. I haven't seen much of her, and John and I decided to take her out for her ninety-fourth birthday breakfast with Cara over the weekend. This worked out and pleased her. We enjoyed the time together. She expects to sell her home of over sixty years, and will move away to be closer to one of her daughters in Ohio. After the last couple of years, I know it will be best for her to be close to that part of her family.

Our friend Tony stopped by one evening to leave some reading material for John. After a short chat we decided to go out with him and Maryann, for an impromptu supper out. We shared all the demanding details of each other's lives and had a few laughs in the process. As if the holidays aren't crazy enough, we all were going through tough times. *Friends are great levelers and their support usually makes things more bearable.*

December 9, was another doctor appointment with my oncologist. I was still bothered by side effects from the estrogen blocker medication. My demeanor was fairly anxiety ridden and we agreed to stop the drug I was taking as we had discussed last month. We decided that I would not take anything until January when I would try a second drug. I was hoping to have fewer problems with side effects.

This was also the night of Cara's induction into the National Honor Society. It was a surprisingly touching ceremony and event. Don't ask me why, but I did not expect to be so impressed or delighted by the evening. The other situations in our lives were perhaps taking away from more positive expectations. The school handled the occasion with just the right amount of importance and reverence.

We were very proud of our daughter and each of the other young men and women who had made it into this prestigious group. It certainly was nothing *I* ever came close to accomplishing! This was surprisingly exciting.

It was a busy and big month to be sure. To make things even more interesting I found myself working part-time again. I arrived at the nursing home one day to realize that the receptionist was still out from her vacation. Mom informed me that this woman had fallen and broken her hip just before returning to her job. We went to the front desk and inquired as to how she was doing. The administrator assistant who was covering the desk then asked, "Would you be interested in the job? It is for six-eight weeks while she recovers." Without much thought I responded, "Yes."

After a couple of days of formalities I was working the front desk. It was strange at first for me. It had been a while since I had a job. It seemed to be a win-win for me. I would have a more recent job experience to add to my resume, perhaps another reference, and some small amount of income for this holiday season. I thought Garry might find comfort in knowing I was working part-time right in the building where he was living. It was a small welcomed adventure.

What seemed like an easy job turned out to be much more demanding than I had would have guessed. The holidays made the home frantically busy. Between increased visitors, mail, phone calls, and lots of added packages and flowers—it was hectic. Seeing what goes on daily in a nursing home was insightful. It occurred to me; one large problem is that many people expect a nursing home to be a cross between a hotel and a hospital. In reality it is neither. It is a care facility. Most of the caregivers are not nurses or doctors.

This particular home has a very highly regarded reputation. Even so, in truth, no one who doesn't have to would ever want to live in any nursing home. Living at your own home with appropriate care is ideal, but practically impossible. Truthfully, if Garry was still able to participate socially it might have worked better for him. I was grateful that it was a nice, clean, visitor-friendly place, which made it much easier on us.

As I settled in the job, I realized that it was time for me to find something with more permanence. The staff knew who I was because of my frequent visits during the past six months. Many people would stop by the desk and inquire about my brother and how my parents were holding up. Often they would comment about what a pleasure our family was.

There was one odd moment when an employee and I got to talking. I told her about my breast cancer crisis and about my brother having ALS, and added that my son was having a second knee surgery in a couple of weeks. She had a rather perplexed expression and asked me, "Do you ever ask yourself why all these terrible things are happening to *you* and your family?" I was really shocked at this comment and it took me a long time to get it out of my head. How insensitive. It was extremely awkward, but I chalked the comment up to being a clumsy mistake and for once bit my tongue.

The Human Resources Administrator has told me she will keep me in mind if something else comes along—though it would be nice if it was that easy, I was not counting on that. At least, the experience had given me more confidence about working again, which was good.

TOUGH ENDS AND
ROUGH BEGINNINGS

My cousin's wife Carol hosted a holiday party this year at a restaurant. Thoughtfully she selected a spot in New Jersey, where Mom, Vicki and I could attend more easily. I remember last year declining any party as I was germ phobic while I was in the middle of chemo treatments.

This year Carol pointed out that it was more "important not to miss the occasion again." It seemed like a difficult request, but I also thought it was the right thing to do. We agreed on December 18, at a fine-dining spot where we had a private room that was just perfect. How lovely! This was a no-work treat.

Though we all were thinking of Garry and how much he would have loved being with us, we barely spoke about him. Everyone tried to keep things as light as possible. Garry was unaware that this gathering was taking place; I knew this was tough on my Mom and Irwin. I believed it was important to spend this holiday time together. We had not seen my Aunt Betty, her children or their families much and this evening was sweet.

The next week was predictably busy. Thankfully my Christmas shopping went reasonably smooth earlier on. I was comfortably prepared and ready. My week included a couple of work days, which meant a bit more juggling on my end, but things seemed fairly calm. Christmas day we expected to be joined by Mom, Irwin, Vicki, Paul, Jen and Dave. John's family all had other plans.

Our Dempsey Christmas morning was just as we like it. In the morning, we wait for Anne to arrive to open the gifts, and then share a breakfast together. Our gift exchange left everyone happy and content.

Anne and Dave were sent home after breakfast because she was not feeling well. I asked them to come back later rather than to hang around spreading germs. The concern was that we might make everyone else sick. Avoiding spreading any illness was now even higher on my list. Also, Cara was out of sorts and coming down with what must have been a stomach virus. My sissy hates being near anyone who is not feeling well. Great, we were Germ-Central; this was definitely not going to be a hit! We tried our best to keep up a healthy appearance. Oy!

It all went fine. It was this quiet group that we needed to spend our day with. We all sorely missed Garry. I was pleased to have my sister, Paul and Jen join us. Vicki and I were comfortable and happy to share the day together as always.

There was a big storm expected for Monday. As I had not seen Garry in a couple of days, I was determined to head over for a visit before it got terribly nasty out on Sunday. I headed out early and met up with Garry's friend Linda who came every Sunday morning for a visit. Mom and Irwin were already there as well. We all told my brother not to worry if no one returned for a day or so because of the storm.

Linda has been an incredible friend to Garry, coming faithfully every week to the nursing home. Until this time I never met her in all the years of their friendship. Garry was not easily engaged this day and we were all concerned about him. Linda spoke of how my brother helped her cope with the frustrations of being a stay-at-home mom of two active young children. She said, "When I needed to talk to someone, he was always willing to listen and cheer me up. Believe me Garry did a lot more for me than I did for him." Linda was sincere and her loyalty was impressive. Mom and Irwin always looked forward to her visits.

By that night, I felt a bad cold coming on. The next couple of days were awful for me. Against my better judgment and my boss's insistence, I made it to work on Wednesday. Then, John was sick by mid-week. New Year's Eve was spent recuperating and even quieter than is our custom. My husband longs for a loud and trashy New Year's event and I always want the opposite. I dislike the whole evening and the anticipation that it brings. There was no choice this year and it was not my fault. Ah, 2011. I am afraid to even think what this year will bring.

Actually I wrote out and sent my Christmas cards after the holiday. That was a task that I thought to forgo this year. Then I managed to put together a letter that felt comfortable to send along with our cards.

An old friend who moved to Florida found Cara on Facebook and inquired about how I was doing. She was happy to finally make contact in this way. Well, since I had just coincidentally sent her another Christmas card and letter, I left the communication at that. I just wasn't sure how to react to her message. A card that said "Get well" or "Thinking of You" would have been greatly appreciated by me. Still, I was glad to hear from her now. Hey, I also miss plenty of opportunities to do the right thing—plenty!

I heard from Maryann, who brought us dreadfully disturbing news that our neighbor has been diagnosed with a very serious health issue. The amount of acute problems is really overwhelming. I sent a note to his wife Dee (she left me the lovely friend-ornament in my mailbox). Now, she knows we are aware of their situation and that they were in our thoughts. She called me days later and said that her husband was undergoing an alternative therapy. As I would have expected she was optimistic and positive.

Someone really deserves a miracle; I am thinking of several people I care deeply about. My husband says, "We have reached the age when these types of problems happen more frequently."

The beginning of January brought the announcement that hospice felt Garry had reached a kind of status quo. They could not continue providing the care he had been receiving. Garry did not seem particularly attached to the caregiver. Even so, we all knew he was getting better care. It seemed almost heartless that this determination was made.

The current hospice-aide was a doll. Mostly, she could offer only to clean my brother well. That was huge. She talked to him and dressed him for the day. No matter how he growled at her, she always accepted his frustrations and met them with a warm smile. We had several caregivers before her arrival and she seemed special to us. We felt badly that this particular aide was being taken off Garry's case in about two weeks.

This was a wild week. Besides my work days, Anne had been given short notice that court was scheduled again on Wednesday morning. Then, Keith's second surgery on his knee was two days later on January 7.

Anne was ready to testify and get the case behind her. John, Dave and I accompanied her to court. We were there several hours. Our daughter told her side of the story very clearly, controlled, and with the confidence of the truth.

The defendant was far less credible as his sleaziness was fairly palpable throughout his testimony. The defense lawyer suggested in a roundabout fashion that Anne's motive was actually to have another court case. The implication was she would likely sue this same person in the future to receive a monetary reward. He insisted on repeatedly asking her to point out her other attorney. It actually provided some silent levity, because the defense lawyer was referring to John, who wore a suit to court. It appeared the defense attorney was the only one who did not understand that John was Anne's father and not her attorney.

Anne is of Mexican heritage, and looks nothing like either John or me. Luckily she is not sensitive; our biracial, interfaith family makes all our skin a bit thicker at times. None of us offered any explanation. After many nasty and harsh comments to Anne throughout the morning, we quite enjoyed his mistake and discomfort. John may have clued him in by taking and holding my hand as we continued to watch him make his point.

The defendant was established in the community and familiar to our daughter before the incident because he was a bank customer where she worked. He was also not young. Those facts made her feel more uncomfortable about reporting what had taken place. Anne's main concern was that he should not inflict harm on anyone else. This was a first step to seeing that he might be stopped. Wow! It was not easy. Anne did her duty and I hoped this outcome will help her. She was still obviously rocked by this incident.

In the end, the Judge charged the defendant guilty and gave him a fine. More importantly this man has a blemish on his record. If there is a next time, he will receive a stronger punishment. That is *all* Anne wanted. This was a great service to the community and we were proud of our daughter. I am thankful it went this way. We were all relieved.

Keith's surgery on Friday was more involved and extensive than we had expected. After several hours he had a new ACL and some other repair to his knee. The doctor told us that this was a weight-bearing recovery; it might be a little easier but recovery would be as long as the first one.

We brought Keith home the same day. He was not comfortable and later he bled so heavily that we called the doctor. The covering surgeon said, "It is normal after surgery to the bone to bleed substantially." It was upsetting to me because it did so extremely heavily for quite a while. Of course, Keith was relatively calm, but John was definitely concerned as well. We all carefully watched the situation until it appeared to be under control. What a week!

SURPRISES

This was Keith's semester break and he was stuck at home and in bed most of the next five or six days. He used rented equipment to move the leg properly and to strengthen it again as prescribed right away. He wanted to return to his apartment, his job, and his last semester at school as soon as possible.

Keith's follow-up appointment was on John's birthday, January 14. I drove him to this appointment as he certainly was unable to get there on his own. He was on crutches and with all the snow and ice it was even more challenging to get around.

The doctor was pleased. Surgeons openly admire their own work, in my experience. Later we arranged for "handicapped parking" at college for when Keith returned to driving. This made me feel better, as he needed crutches for a while. Carrying all his school paraphernalia was tricky enough; running for buses and managing long distances in bad weather would be worse. We lucked out, and for a price the issue was solved.

Next, we ate lunch together and Keith informed me that Anne, Cara and he had bought John a special gift. He was bound by a promise not to tell me what it was. Well, that made me very suspicious and quickly got the best of me. I asked him to tell me. Finally, I told him to ask Anne if I could go in on it also; something made me certain it was expensive. I had no ideas or time to buy John anything. I knew he was not even expecting a gift from me today.

Keith did some rapid texting and was given the go-ahead to tell me what "it" was, and what my share in this "amazing surprise" was going to be. They had bought John a Stratocaster guitar. It was a second-hand treasure. Dave and Keith had heard John say he would like to have one someday, and they were sure he would love the one they found. They also have heard me say, "No more guitars!" They worried about my reaction.

I actually thought this was a great, special gift and I also knew John deserved this. It was a pleasure for me to have money I had earned recently to contribute to the birthday gift. We were all excited to surprise him later.

After dinner and before dessert we gave John his gift. Anne and Dave confused him with a fake present first. Then, Cara popped into the room pretending she was playing the blue and white, sexy beauty, the real gift. There will be lots more "rock'n" at our house from now on! John was really excited! This was the best gift he has ever received and he was delighted.

Keith was headed back to school as semester break was over. I was concerned about his recovery. Basically, John reminded me that our son was able to take care of himself and I should not worry about him. Yeah, that would never happen!

Keith's roommate drove Keith's car back to school. The car was loaded to the max. Both boys packed their returning clothes, food, games and toys, along with Keith's rehabilitation devices, and they were off. We were fairly sure that by having the car with him, Keith would be back on the road probably sooner than not. He did have school, a job, and more physical therapy ahead.

A surprise gift came today in the form of a check. Contact with my dad's cousin, Debby, in recent years has been reduced to my annual holiday letter. This gesture felt very important because it was unexpected. I sent her a letter immediately and thanked her. Recently Mom and she have been speaking regularly by phone. Debby is quite interested in Garry's situation and about the rest of us. This was a welcome change from the medical bills that keep arriving.

—ᵚ—

Garry was assigned a new hospice organization after about two weeks. We were all grateful, as he was not cleaned as well during this period. It was quite apparent that he was continuing to decline. The new arrangement allowed for an aide every day, which seemed to be a great advantage. However, the aides changed often and arrived at different times. Once in a while they did not come. This was a little disconcerting, especially for my brother who needed consistency and dependability.

Thank God people were stopping by to spend a little time with Garry. His friend Greg and his family would come by regularly. Greg and his wife Barbara had known my brother since Garry was a young boy in summer camp and they were counselors there. Linda was there like clockwork on Sundays. Some group home residents and staff, and a couple of his work friends and Vicki's friend Michelle occasionally stopped by in the evenings. Mom and Irwin were devoted to being with him every day.

There were other people who we did not know about because Garry could not tell us.

Garry was fortunate he was so loved and admired. As difficult as it was to see him this way, everyone wanted to be there for him. People came despite the bad winter weather. There were less visits though as my brother became harder to engage.

On work days, I only had my fifteen-minute break and my lunch half-an-hour for visiting Garry. Sometimes, I would visit before work started when I was early and he was awake. After work was over for the day I never went back upstairs to visit him. That was his dinner time and he would have insisted on my staying to feed him. It was also the time of day when he did a great deal more choking. Earlier on, I would be there at that time and I found it too disturbing. My mission at 5:00 was to get home and make dinner for my family. I was always uncomfortable on my drive home.

At this point, Garry's speech was very limited and hard to understand. He rarely said more than, "some drink" or "ice cream" or "to bed." He also had acquired one strange vice. Whenever he said goodbye to Mom and Irwin he would say, "f-u-c-k y-o-u" with a hint of a smile. Thank goodness he said it softly because *that* was pretty clear most times. There were times that you did not hear him say the words. But you could see him move his lips enough so that you definitely knew what he meant. There was usually a hint of humor that he conveyed with a glance. You sensed it brought him some satisfaction; that almost made you feel better, too. He also had taken a shot at Vicki and I as the opportunity presented itself. He was probably so tortured by not being able to communicate that it may have pleased him momentarily to "give it to us." At least, it was short if not sweet! This did not upset or offend us.

Garry also cursed the aides and staff out regularly. This was unfortunate. For some reason these words were the clearest in his present repertoire. Perhaps they were easier to say and to be understood. They definitely communicated his anger and discomfort. Otherwise, we just got to know his requests and could usually figure out what he was asking for. We guessed about what he might want to say, and told him about things we thought he would want to hear.

Often, he seemed less present. I never thought his mind was affected by anything other than the anguish of pain and frustration from the ALS. It had robbed him of movement and communication. ALS affects the nerves, which eventually leave the muscles unable to work; the prison this disease creates is completely cruel. The difference between even a "yes" and "no" was hard to distinguish. Finally, we would ask him to smile if he meant "yes." This was a small movement he made with usually his right cheek. I had heard people say that it often comes down to blinking as the last form of communication.

An aide got very annoyed in front of me one afternoon. She turned to Garry sternly and raised her voice reminding him, "I am a Christian woman and won't stand for that language." She made me nervous, because most of the other aides seemed to handle this much better. There was a tone in what she said that conveyed a warning. I was uncomfortable. Maybe she wanted me to know this was unacceptable to her.

How could these people understand how out of character all this really was? Hey, I'm sure this is a tough, demanding and often nasty job. For the most part the staff appeared caring and efficient.

There were rarely enough people to quickly attend to all the requests and needs at any given time. We still felt Garry was very lucky to be where he was. This was a highly respected place with an outstanding reputation. Evaluating any residents' point of view is difficult as their condition may make their comfort and satisfaction nearly impossible.

THE BEST MEDICINE

Cara was very busy at school now working on the play. The play this year is *"No, No, Nanette"* As usual the dedication and commitment was impressive. For the parents it was not much less. The practice schedule was demanding. We knew it would be worth it in the end. Cara had less time for visiting Garry while she was juggling school work and practices. Now and then we got her over for a short visit. Garry adores her and missed her. Anne had cold after cold, and was not by to see her uncle frequently either. Keith was mostly at school and his visits were few.

In the meantime, I started my new estrogen blocker medication. It was worse than the first one, as it made me nauseous and then chilled for hours each night. I knew that I would stop using this one as soon as possible. I had an appointment soon and I would talk things over then with my doctor.

Laura's husband has been receiving encouraging reports lately, which we are so happy to hear. Our neighbor seems to be doing well, too. All the same problems are still being dealt with, but for now they were somewhat under control.

Cara is a high school junior and is looking forward to her Junior Prom. She asked me to make a rare trip to a NY mall on Sunday, where she would be able to buy the perfect prom dress. The new thing is: Buy the dress, and then post a picture on your computer to keep anyone else from purchasing the exact same one. OMG, really? Well, after five full shopping hours we purchased a beautiful navy blue gown. It was actually a great day. I was thrilled to see how happy Cara was with her find. Her amazing red hair and the dress color looked great and the style was just right for her. This major task was taken care of. Now, she could relax knowing this is done. All we had to do was get the dress hemmed and accessorized. No sweat, we had plenty of time for that.

The good part about journaling is that I can appreciate more of what is happening. Life has a funny way of balancing out a bit. My project makes me feel a little guilty because of the time that I give to it.

My job came to end by mid-February. The receptionist returned recovered and ready to reclaim her position. She had always been very sweet to us and I was glad to see her doing well. She was kind enough to thank me for helping out and mentioned how much she liked the new directory I had designed for the front desk. I appreciated that acknowledgment. It felt odd to rejoin the ranks of the unemployed so soon. I had just started to feel comfortable about the job. Actually in my shallow list of recent employment positions it may rank fairly high.

For the record, once employed there and after learning more about this home we never brought in anything else for my brother to eat. Surely, it would have cost me my job to do so. Now I had to respect the rules; of course, that is not to say they made complete sense to me. Oh dear! I would have loved making Garry happier with outside food he might enjoy. I told him as an employee I had more of a responsibility to obey the rules. I think he understood that position and was tolerant as it related to my job.

Meanwhile, Mom and Irwin were not giving in to the wear and tear of being with Garry. We were all worried about the toll this was having on them in particular. It was terrible for everyone, but they are not young people anymore and this schedule was grueling. We all continued to stop by as often as possible.

One afternoon in particular, Laura and I came to visit and we were trying everything possible to bring Garry a little cheer. Finally, after he requested to be back in bed and when he was settled we got very silly. Our jokes, smiles and hugs were not getting it done.

I suggested we sing him some of his favorite songs. Laura followed my lead immediately. We conjured up the tunes *Going to the Chapel, Rambling Rose, Rhinestone Cowboy, Mona Lisa* and *The Lion Sleeps Tonight*. Now, that interesting group of tunes was specifically my brother's all-time favorites.

Each song brought recognition along with a big smile and a silent laugh. We had not seen this from Garry in a very long time. It was so funny, really. Mom came in on it toward the end, making our trio perfect. We all together, definitely had the worst voices ever! It was pitiful the poor guy was subjected to so much already; we were almost torturing him more than entertaining him. I believe he did find genuine enjoyment in those few minutes, and it was well worth making fools out of ourselves for that. I will always treasure that memory.

Anne took me to my doctor in New York again on February 2. After describing my side effects from the second pill, I chose to return to the first one again. This estrogen blocker medication is apparently quite important and my doctor was adamant about me taking it. The third choice of medicines comes with risks I am unwilling to take.

After we finished in the city Anne wanted to see her Uncle Garry, who she had not visited in a while. She was disturbed by the obvious changes taking place with him. She seemed glad that we stopped by together to spend time with him.

Ginny, Colette, Diane and I have been constantly texting to update each other. John and I managed to crash over Ginny's one evening and we had a good time with her and Greg. Mostly, my visits with my brother were the focus of my time.

It was later in February and the play was just about to open. The rehearsals were intense and I was starting to get nervous. John and I were taking Mom and Irwin to opening night. Anne and Dave joined us and at the last minute Maryann called and came along, too. Earlier this afternoon Cara was so unglued we thought this year's play might not go well. We wanted to make sure it was OK before we invited the rest of our crew. We are hoping this was just stage fright.

The show was terrific. Cara was hilarious! Her roll was as the snarky, malcontent maid. It was not a big part, though with each enormous laugh she drew from the audience it grew larger. The show was adorable and Cara was wonderful. It was the best time; Even Grandma and Grandpa were thrilled. It was hard to imagine anything could make them really happy at this point in time. This performance was just the ticket!

All the actors put in a fine effort and several were outstanding. Tonight, Cara was the bright star! We swelled with pride; it was the most amazing feeling. Of course, now I had to start rounding up others to see the play the rest of that weekend and the next.

Out of seven performances, I missed only one. We have two casts of leads. A number of leads switch with their ensemble counterpart. It is such a treat to see the growth of each person as the years have gone by. Cara's buddies all did a super job and it was a blast. *This was just what the doctor should have ordered—lots of fun!*

The memory of that first night will be forever embossed in our hearts. We brought a number of people to see the remaining performances. Everyone was impressed and pleasantly surprised. All the hard work and sacrifices paid off—yay!!

OUR SADDEST DAY

I had started to use the first medication again and unfortunately experienced all the original issues. The sleep-aid medication, which I try to use sparingly to tolerate the blocker, does help. We will see how this goes. I am trying to appreciate the necessity of the estrogen blocker. The months of April and May will bring lots of different doctor appointments and certainly more discussion on this subject.

Mom's birthday on March 2 was tricky and we felt despite Garry's condition it should not be overlooked. Irwin suggested a dinner out on Sunday. Mom, Irwin, Vicki, Paul, Jen, John and I had a delicious meal together to mark Mom's birthday. It was the best we could manage.

It seemed obvious that Garry was more remote, thinner (hard to believe) and weaker each time I saw him. He stayed in bed more of the day. Even almost reclined in his wheeled hospital chair he did not want to stay in areas outside his bedroom for any length of time.

There was a small and unusual stretch of about four days where I did not go to see Garry. Laura and I had planned to visit on Thursday. Severe rain reports made us cancel that plan. Laura is almost a half-hour from our home and I think her area is more of a problem than ours generally. We both have flooding concerns and wet basements in heavy rain situations. Laura and Artie were leaving for a rare one-week vacation on Saturday. Laura said she would visit as soon as she could when they got back.

When I returned to see my brother on Monday, March 7, I was horrified to notice Garry's condition had worsened. His swallowing was much more difficult. His reflex muscles were not working right anymore. We gave him his cranberry juice and ice cream like always, but we had to tell him to swallow what was placed in his mouth. That seemed to take a huge effort. I felt this was a serious and frightening development. The week was awful. A day or two later the nurses and aides were remarking that his appetite had also diminished. How unbearable! This went from very little to almost none.

My plan was to definitely return on the weekend with John and the girls. It occurred to me that Laura and I should not have postponed our visit last week. She certainly had done more than I could ever have asked or expected of her!

201

Note: this was also the week of the horrendous and devastating earthquake in Japan—it felt as though "bad things" were in the air.

John, Cara and I went to see my brother Sunday afternoon. Anne met us after a little while and I was glad she made it. Mom and Irwin were there and looked exhausted. It was grim visiting with barely any response from my brother.

People who had become friendly with us and others familiar with who we were came by and expressed their concerns, trying to offer comfort. Everyone felt what was happening to Garry. Alex and his daughter Ellen were with us much of the time.

When we left the home I turned to my family and said, "You saw Uncle Garry for the last time today." The girls both seemed surprised with the statement. They were glad they came to see him. In my heart I thought it would only be a day two more before Garry was gone.

Usually I arrived at Garry's at about 12:30. This morning I called Mom early to tell her that my front yard tree was scheduled to be removed in a few minutes, at 8:30. Afterward I would go to my brother's right away. She informed me that the home called her already to say he would likely pass away this morning so they were heading there very early. This was no surprise to me.

I let Vicki know what was happening and she planned to join us as soon as she could. When I got to Garry's room Mom was there by his side. Garry was on oxygen breathing laboriously and not able to show us any sign of consciousness. Vicki joined us and then had to leave a while, but returned later.

All day long, people came in and out. Some we knew over these past nine months and some we had no connection with. Alex and a few other closer acquaintances were quietly sitting vigil nearby. Some people stepped into Garry's room and would make a comment or offered a glance that said just as much.

A few persons actually made me less comfortable as they seemed to be almost intrusive and cold. Most we did not mind. Some offered information about Garry's condition. The skin around joint areas looked bruised and his face was paled and graying.

There was one particular aide who stepped in later in the afternoon that I had taken great exception to being with us. She had always been a concern because my brother would get so agitated and disturbed by her presence. We could not accuse her of anything. Yet, his reaction was strong around her and it was upsetting. She would always respond to him by saying something like, "Garry, you are my little baby. Garry, you are OK, you are my baby, right?"

Garry never liked to hear condescending statements and maybe that is all it was—we will never know. We had requested she not be assigned to him, but this was not always possible. She also gave me the creeps, and her presence was not acceptable to me today!

Unfortunately, the brand new hospice person had also just arrived. After tolerating the aide's quiet and bizarre presence for a number of minutes, I announced that they would have to leave and give us some privacy. It was Mom, Garry's regular nurse, the new hospice person, the strange aide and me with Garry. Mom looked at me in disbelief and said, "Don't be that way." I insisted, and we did not discuss it further.

I think Mom was afraid that we might not be able to be with Garry at some point later. She did not want to leave her son with any problems and no defense. Maybe I am way off.

A couple of minutes later, I went down the hall to explain and apologize for being so curt. The regular nurse had obviously, already spoken with the new hospice aide and filled her in. The hospice RN was also in the little office when I stepped in to talk with them. They suggested we talk to Garry about it being OK to leave us, and tell him that we will all be fine. We could say how much we loved him and knew he fought very hard, but that he did not have to do that anymore. Anyway, I think that is an accurate summary.

They said, "Hearing is the last thing to go before dying. Even at this stage he might receive some of the messages." They said, "Sometimes, people need to hear these words before they are able to let go."

Garry never spoke about being ready or wanting to die. We never offered these ideas out of concern it would cause him any more upset or fear. *Being a family of vague faith makes the whole process of death much more uncertain and uncomfortable,* I think. My mother was definitely not going to digest hearing this well. It left me in a real quandary.

Anne surprised us with her company which caused me additional worry as I was not sure how she would handle all this. Vicki returned and joined us. Later the social worker, who knew Garry for a long time, came in the room. I liked this man and respected him for the many efforts he extended to our family. He and his wife actually worked for the group home organization Garry lived at for some time. His wife had come by to visit my brother in the nursing home and she gave him a green stuffed frog holding a heart for Valentine's Day.

Today, the social worker wanted to see my brother before he left work for the day and a week's vacation. Eric was glassy-eyed as he spoke with us, and I could see he understood Garry would be gone when he came back to work again. He asked me if we spoke to my brother about the things which the nurses had already suggested. He said, "Garry's definitely fighting to stay with us and it might help him to let go."

The hours passed. Finally Irwin insisted that he take Mom home and that they would return when needed or very early the next day. Mom wavered and then decided to leave knowing we were staying later into the evening. Irwin felt strongly that they needed to take care of eating and getting a little sleep for the wearing day ahead.

Shortly after they left, I leaned into Garry and stroked his head and arm. I told him, "Garry, you don't need to struggle anymore. We want you to just be at peace now." We told him how much he was loved and how great he had always been to us and everyone he knew. These messages were delivered over and over again as the time passed.

Around 11:00 I encouraged my sister to go home. Garry was exactly as he had been for many hours. Anne and I told her we would stay through the night, and call her if anything happened. Vicki was under a lot of added business pressure because of an important early morning appointment she was handling for one of her associates, who also had an emergency.

Anne, of course, was not going to allow any negotiation as to her leaving her uncle or me. We sat together talking and touching him lovingly throughout the night. During this time staff came and went mostly with little if anything even spoken.

One unknown woman kept returning. She would tell us to be sure to speak to and touch Garry. She became a bit meddling to me; her interest felt strange. I am not sure what she was up to. Was she caring or did she want us to pray? I don't know. It felt as if she wanted to be right there when he left us. Maybe I misunderstood her? My mind was racing around every corner.

Before 2:00 in the morning we noticed an irregular and erratic difference in Garry's breathing. At this point, I phoned Mom and Vicki to let them know that the end was close. I told my sister about the change and suggested we would see her later in the day. Mom and Irwin were coming as soon as they could. Anne and I watched reluctantly in disbelief as Garry took his last breaths and slipped away minutes later on March 15, 2011.

The same staff person returned immediately again. Maybe these people think you want their company at this time. Wrong.

My greatest consolation is that Garry did not choke to death and that he was not alone, without family at his side. It seemed to me for some time now, that he was afraid of the first, and likely dreaded the second. He labored, but he did seem peaceful today and I was grateful for that.

Anne was just wonderful about "being there" for her Uncle Garry and me. It was good that we were able to share this hugely important experience together. Mom and Irwin arrived soon after that. Mom had a hard time staying in the room, so we left after a short while.

This may sound strange, but Mom and Irwin suggested that we all needed to take care of ourselves now. As is our traditional remedy, we knew where to head. It was around 4:00 in the morning when the four of us sat wiped out, saddened and still in disbelief over an early and needed breakfast in a local diner. We missed Garry already.

Sorrow and Joy

om and Irwin had told us a while back that Garry would be cremated, which is my preference also. Irwin felt strongly that he wanted to sit Shiva right away. Mom seemed OK with this plan. Then they decided on a memorial arrangement at the nursing home chapel in the near future.

The obituary they submitted for the next day's publication only said that the memorial would be announced at a later date. Mom seemed intent on expecting only the people who were steadily in touch with us or Garry to be interested in attending. I was certain his connections were vast and more people would want to pay their last respects to him.

John and I ran out Tuesday morning to pick up items that would be helpful for Mom's house over the next few days. Oddly enough, as we drove I noticed a car driving on my right side traveling perfectly even with us. I was in the passenger seat and it was a few seconds before I realized what it was. It was an empty, black hearse and the name on its door was the funeral home where my Dad had gone. Weird? It was a sign—I felt my Dad was telling me that he was with Garry.

A number of people came to Mom's house over the next few days. My Aunt Betty came with her son Eric and his daughter Alex. Her other son Peter and his wife Carol and their son Doug came too. We were glad they were all there with us.

My friends Ginny and Greg, Colette, Dan and Diane came by as I might have expected. Of course, Laura was still away and uninformed. Some former neighbors heard and came though it had been a very long time since we had been in touch. Vicki's in-laws and mine also were quick to share this condolence time.

There were other friends and acquaintances that imparted sweet memories and recollections with us. Mostly, the word about the Shiva did not reach many others. Garry's work associates, group home people, camp friends and more did not know about this opportunity to join us. Since we are not religious, and there was no immediate funeral service and the memorial date had not been announced, many people were not sure what to expect.

Friday morning before I headed to Mom's for the last day of the Shiva, I received a call. Colette told me her mom passed away earlier that morning. Colette actually had taken her entire family to visit Etta this day. Her mom slipped away surrounded by the devoted family who loved her. It seemed meant to be that they were all there at her side.

I was not shocked to hear of her passing. However, it was strange to think we lost both Garry and Etta within days of one another this week! My friend had tried to hold on to her mother for a long time now. Understandably she seems to be experiencing disbelief that this had finally happened.

My thoughts and prayers are with their family. I too, am saddened by Etta's passing; I am very glad for the time we spent together this past year. Thursday evening the following week, John and I attended the wake. We saw their family, some of whom we remembered and some who we never knew. John had not seen Colette since her dad passed.

Friday morning was Colette's mother's funeral. A large group of Etta's nursing home staffers and residents were in attendance. My friend and her brother spoke lovingly of their mom at the church. I felt good knowing how important this tribute was for my friend. I attended the repast, but left early.

—\~—

This was a day of extremes and I needed to switch gears. The Junior Prom was this evening and Cara had a hair appointment. I left the repast in a hurry to get to the salon on time. My daughter was calmer than I expected; I was more nervous. I wanted Cara to be happy with how she looked and to have a good time.

Cara was beautiful and her date very handsome. They both appeared happy and confident. My mom and Irwin came by briefly to see their granddaughter off. They were worn out and missing their usual oomph, but they would not miss an opportunity to share this little bit of the event with us. They have done this with each of our children at every prom. Anne came home after Cara left with her date and his parents. They met friends for a huge photo shoot that always takes place prior to the main event.

Anne and I followed to see the mayhem happening across town firsthand. There were three party buses waiting to transport the large number of prom-goers. Extra people who wanted to see them before they left filled the streets.

The buses had to park several streets away. All I could do was wonder how Cara would walk in the five-inch heels she had on and never broke in. My suspicion is that they are not for walking in at all. One of the parents wisely poured a group of girls into their van and drove them to their bus. Hooray! Anne and I would have helped but we were parked too far away to do the same.

They were off. It was fun to see our babies all "grown up" tonight. Everything seemed fine. Oh, the things a single day can bring!

ARRANGEMENTS AND REMEMBRANCES

Mom received random visitors over the course of the next few days. It was very rewarding to hear how much my brother had meant to all of them. The plan was to hold Garry's memorial on April 3. This happened to be the date of *my* Dad and Mom's wedding anniversary. That felt like a good omen to me.

Mom depended on "word of mouth" to let people know about the arrangements. She was so concerned that the home was not prepared, or interested in a large crowd and she discouraged some people from attending. Some she asked not to bring additional family members, or asked others to only select a small number from a group (such as his coworkers). I was concerned about this effort on her part, and I understood this was all very difficult for her. We asked the home's Rabbi to preside over the service.

The Rabbi knew that we were not a religious family. Perhaps his cleric experiences in the Armed Forces have made him more tolerant. I had become familiar with the Rabbi's casual and accessible manner, and was certain he would be comfortable with the memorial we wanted have for my brother.

We had a planned group of speakers to say something about Garry during the service. Irwin insisted on being the first to ulogize my brother. I definitely wanted to speak. Mom's friend Joan wanted to read something she had written. Mom asked Garry's dear friend Linda, his nursing home social worker Eric, and his former work counselor Denise to deliver speeches. Irwin's son Alan also planned some additional touches. This seemed like a very personal way for us to have a small tribute to Garry, and it was scheduled approximately three weeks after he passed away.

The date was not good for a few people we would have so liked to join us. It was impossible to arrange a perfect day for everyone. Anne was leaving for a ten-day vacation to Texas and delaying for her return was not wise. As it was, this wait felt strange.

Alan came from Colorado on Thursday before the memorial, which was to be on Sunday. He planned to read his wife's written tribute to Garry and say a few words of his own.

Admittedly, I was dissatisfied that Alan was to end the speeches. After all, Irwin earned the right to be first by his relationship and his devotion to my brother. Also, his poor hearing might have made his speech awkward if Irwin did not hear clearly what had been said before him. However, Alan ending this important occasion did not seem as appropriate to me. Garry has natural siblings who have adored him for the past fifty-five years. It was uncomfortable for me to decide how important this was going to be for me to accept.

I decided not to make a request to alter this plan. I thought maybe I would have a difficult time listening to everyone else and not get through my speech without being a wreck. I did not want to cause hard feelings and then "blow it" by falling apart. There was no doubt that we all meant well; and I was aware that I was becoming anxiety ridden.

In the meantime, Laura came home to our sad news. It certainly was not unexpected. Artie was not feeling well and there were more concerns on their end. She was sure she would be at the memorial; although she had to be at work later that afternoon. Artie would try to attend. I also had told Laura about Colette's mom, who she knew fairly well. My girlfriends would see each other for the first time in many years. I knew that was not a problem for either of them. Laura was very supportive and I was glad she was back. My friend has been through so much also. We are all worn out.

I was totally unnerved generally. It was very important to me that I do a good job honoring my sweet brother. Since public speaking is not "my thing" I knew I would definitely need to write my speech out carefully. No lie, I typed away and made additions and corrections for days. It became an obsession with me. I read and reread my piece. Anything I stumbled on or started to cry over was modified until it felt comfortable and right. Finally, I felt that I was ready to share my carefully chosen thoughts.

Vicki and I had talked and agreed we wanted to celebrate Garry for the extraordinary person he was. John also suggested that I make some funny comments, as Garry would be happy about that. That would make this homage much easier on all. Actually I was comfortable that I had covered all the bases and we were all in agreement. My hope was that I had paid my brother a well-earned tribute. The order of the speeches did not matter in the end.

There was a funny coincidence on the day before the Memorial; we read the newspaper on Saturday morning at home over breakfast as usual.

In the magazine section was a question about Goldie Hawn's middle initial "G"? The answer was that she had a special and funny Uncle Garry who passed away and she was given his initial. His name was spelled, "G-A-R-R-Y" with two "Rs", which is a much less common spelling. It was a sign; seeing my brother's name in the newspaper today made me feel good.

On April 3, Irwin shared deeply personal feelings about his reluctance to get involved with my mother years ago. Irwin explained, "As a special education teacher, I understood the challenges fairly well. Upon our first meeting, I saw how special Garry was and knew that there would never be any problem there."

This was a very honest story and also a tremendous compliment to my brother. I also liked that he remembered that Garry started every day expecting to find some fun.

Next, my reading went fine. My delivery was respectable and even my few jokes went over comfortably. I meant every word. Garry would have liked what I said and that was important to me.

Mom's dear friend Joan read a short and lovely tribute she wrote in her sincere and well-crafted style. We all were glad that she and Marvin were with us today.

Linda gave a heartfelt speech detailing the impressive accomplishments of, both, my father and brother in the Arc organization throughout the years. She expressed beautifully how much Garry's friendship had meant to her and described him as a devoted and special friend. She also mentioned he would often call her at 8:30 in the evening just to say, "I love you."

The other speakers added lovely thoughts and remembrances as well. It was truly comforting and just right. Everyone genuinely conveyed a deep and loving admiration for my brother and an understanding that he was unique and irreplaceable. There was a shared feeling that we all needed to celebrate his life, and not lament his passing.

Lastly, Alan spoke of how much of an inspiration Garry had been for him and his wife and their special needs child. They appreciated the hope that my brother's life gave to them. He read a piece written by his wife. Then he told some personal stories of Garry's ease and ability to be open and loving.

After we all were finished the Rabbi spoke minimally about Garry. We were reminded to continue as Garry had done, and carry out kindnesses in his memory each day. All this turned out to be a perfect tribute to the person Garry was. It was a great acknowledgment of the love he shared with so many.

Outside the synagogue we continued to enjoy chatting with those who chose to stay and offer their condolences and recollections over the luncheon my mother had arranged. Many people remarked that once Garry made a friend—he made a friend for life. This time was very comforting. Apparently one compliment my brother did shower on a number of women in his life was this one: "I love you, like a sister." Yep, lots of the gals I spoke to could swear they had a brother Garry, too.

GARRY REMEMBERED

The following is the speech I delivered at my brother's memorial on April 3, 2011.

Without great detail, I will only say of my brother Garry, that: He was given issues at birth that sent him on a bumpy road as he traveled through life. Watching his first thirty years was especially amazing, as he surpassed all expectations. Once he got going there was no stopping him. Our family and friends were always proud of Garry and each of his successes. Even his small accomplishments were great ones in our eyes. He was truly an inspiration to many of us along his way to becoming an independent, productive and fulfilled person. We were all extraordinarily fortunate to have him in our lives.

Unlike most of us, Garry extended himself and reached out to others all the time. He did that without any real effort. He wasn't just trying to be nice, or trying to make other people happy; he knew it was the way to make himself happy. He was so wise. It was that unconditional affection for people, which made everyone believe that he would always be there for them. He was loving and accessible, easily making you feel special and comfortable around him. Garry was no "master" of many of the ordinary tasks that most people become proficient at. However, what he did well—he did brilliantly. What is so satisfying for us is that we know so many people cared for and loved Garry very much and that people really "got him." To me, Garry was often a nudge and a stubborn little brother. I wish I could say I only loved him and never took him for granted, but that just wasn't true.

Garry will be fondly remembered as a guy who loved women of all ages and constantly showered them with compliments. For the record Mom, Vicki and I received few of those compliments. However, all his nieces and nephews got plenty of unending adoration.

He definitely liked people in general and just loved children. Garry delighted in sharing a joke, especially a quick pun. If he were standing here now, I might say to him: Gee, you drew quite a good crowd today. To which he would reply: Yeah, there are some pretty sketchy people here. He was actually better at this, but you get the point.

We all remember how he thoroughly enjoyed having a bowl of pasta with friends, going to a social event, or having a little chat on the telephone. He relished making new acquaintances, singing some favorite tunes, watching his old TV reruns, and showing off his superb memory skills. He has probably become famous for his Coca-Cola collection and how much he savored a glass of that, his favorite addition.

In the end, Garry lost far too much. By the time he came to this nursing home, he was challenged in unimaginable ways. The sweet, gentle, funny, little charmer was barely recognizable and he no longer reached out to make new acquaintances. It broke our hearts to know that the caregivers here would never know what a uniquely genuine and incredible person he was. So, for the last nine months, we all acted on his behalf. Yes, even at this stage of his life Garry continued to teach us how to be better versions of ourselves. To their credit Mom and Irwin, who were here every day, certainly became part of the fabric of this nursing home community. In Garry-like fashion, relationships were formed and our world became a little larger and more complete.

Actually I suspect Garry never found any relief, or sense of belonging here. In fact, had he been physically able to, I am sure he would have vamoose-ka-laahed right out the door at his first opportunity! He missed his Fairlawn home and his beloved job so much; and he would have gladly found his way back to both. We all understood this.

On behalf of my family, I would like to thank all the people who came to visit during the last two years in particular. Those of you who came regularly to the nursing home, you will never know how much it meant to Garry and us. A number of you made indescribable efforts we will always remember. But, honestly, all the gestures of kindness, concern and affection toward him are deeply appreciated in ways that we can't adequately express.

We are also indebted to the staff at the nursing home for helping us through this tremendously difficult and sad journey. This is really an exceptional place and we were very fortunate to have been here. A special acknowledgement goes out to Eric, our social worker. Eric, through some act of divine intervention works at the nursing home now, but had known Garry quite a while before he came here. It was a blessing to know Garry had a "friend on the inside" at a time we all needed one.

We miss Garry very much and yet, we are filled with gratitude that his struggle and suffering are over. He took the love of so many with him; and we know he is finally at peace. Personally, I like to think my brother has met my Dad again. I am sure Dad has told Garry how proud he is of his son. In complimentary and sincere style Garry would definitely reply, that he was merely a "chip off the old block."

Garry was a great son, brother, uncle, brother-in-law, nephew, cousin and friend. We are most grateful that he knew how much he was loved. So, we ask you not to remember Garry for his challenges, or his afflictions. Rather, we hope you will think of him as a rare gift and an enormously gracious and wonderful person, who loved us all.

Thank you, for being here today and for sharing this memorial for Garry with us, his family and friends.

It is a guesstimate on my part, that there were about eighty to ninety persons paying their respects on this day. Food and refreshments followed. It was just enough, providing a chance to connect a little more with all who came to be with us and in memory of Garry.

Afterward, Laura and I drove back to my home. She needed to leave about an hour later to go to work at the hospital. Laura was fine, but I could detect extra worry in regards to her husband's health. It was good to have her here with us today. Nothing would have kept her away.

John drove home with his childhood friend Lou, Keith and Cara. Anne, Dave, Mom, Irwin and Alan came back a little while later. We sat around until we were hungry again and ordered some dinner for us all. Anyone else we thought might come home with us had to be elsewhere or was going home to someone sick. It was a long day that went as well as it could have.

My children made me feel especially comfortable regarding my speech. They each expressed that they thought I did a great job and were very supportive. It was important to me; and I loved having their acknowledgment. Honestly, I think the memorial was appropriately personal and sincere. I was pleased everything went well; and I was thankful that the memorial was now behind us.

The next week was spent writing notes to those friends I needed to personally thank for their efforts and condolences. It was an odd time of decompression for me. It all felt very strange on an emotional level.

TIME TO ADJUST

The next weekend, John and I met Vicki and Paul for dinner. It was nice to meet as we had done so often through the years. Yet, it was peculiar not to be together voicing our concerns over what was happening to Garry and Mom and Irwin. It was a mixture of relief and sadness. We knew Mom and Irwin will have an enormous adjustment for a while to come. After all, the nursing home and Garry had been their number one focus every day for over nine months. Not to mention the importance he *always* had on their lives.

Throughout the following days Mom continued to receive calls from people who wanted to pay their respects. There may be a couple of private gatherings which will still happen to honor Garry. His work place and the camp he was associated with for years, both as a camper and an aide, were particularly interested in having some remembrance of him.

Cards and lovely notes from people who knew Garry were still arriving daily. Mom was very touched and overwhelmed by all these gestures. My brother's impact on so many lives was impressive and it is wonderful for us to know about.

Mom and Irwin continue to visit and phone Alex. Irwin and Alex have developed special and rare connection. Their visits will be frequent and I will also continue to see Alex. It is amazing how easily attached you can become to people you have shared even a brief amount of time.

The nursing home is quieter on a number of levels since we stopped having to be there. With pride I can say that we always made attempts to brighten up the place. We were friendly and respectful and very appreciative whenever possible. There was a small community of visitors which became very familiar and close for a number of months; this made the time shared together easier on everyone.

The staff never got to know Garry, but they know our family fairly well now. I am quite sure some regular visitors and a couple of residents miss seeing us around daily. Actually residents and their families are constantly changing; I imagine this is the usual stuff.

Mom and Irwin have started to go through Garry's Coca-Cola collection. Lots of people will be able to keep something as a remembrance. They brought me the clock he had used in his room. We all looked at it so many times each day. I know he always checked out the times we came and went. It's an old fashioned looking red ice-chest clock. It has Coke bottles sitting in ice cubes coming out on top and the trademark white polar bear climbing up the side of it. It is cute and sits on the countertop that goes to our den. I'm glad to have it. Undoubtedly, there will be other mementos added in time.

Anne and Dave went on their ten-day vacation to see her close friends in Texas. Weeks ago, I remember worrying that Anne might be away when Garry passed. At least she was here without any interruption or dilemma at the right time.

Mom and Irwin quietly celebrated their 23rd wedding anniversary on Sunday, April 17. We decided to have a small dinner at home for them, with Vicki and Paul. Jen was in the city; Keith is at school and Anne in Texas. Cara did join us, lucky girl! It turned out well, as it was seriously almost-overlooked. We were glad to be together spontaneously.

Passover, Mom and Irwin went to his niece's home. It was good for them as it provided them with a chance to see Irwin's sister and her husband, who just came up from Florida. I was not ready for this holiday and was happy they were joining their other relatives.

Cara was on spring break this whole week and through Easter. When she was younger I looked forward to that extra time with her. I expect the week will be more about where she is going with her friends. It is still difficult for me to be comfortable with all Cara's friends being new drivers. The girls have planned a trip to NYC on Friday by bus. As fun as that sounds, I will be happy when they are back at home. That's just me.

Our family of five and Dave will be at Tom and Barbara's for Easter this Sunday. Rita, Mary, Anne and I are planning to make many contributions to the food. We are happy to hear that Rita and her children will be with us this year making it more fun. Barbara's children and their families are all also planning to be there this year. Barb's sister and her family will join us as they often do. Wow, it will be a mob!

Vicki and Paul will take Mom and Irwin to a nice restaurant for a holiday meal. So as hard as it is to believe—all the "normal" events and things are falling into place.

Mostly, I have been journaling my head off. It is exciting to return to this endeavor. Fortunately, my notes were invaluable! Last week after many hours at my computer, I had to run to the food store for the tomatoes and cucumbers for that night's salad. When I handed the cashier my store card she read my name off the monitor and said, "What, a great writer's name you have." I looked at her and said, "What?" She repeated herself. How weird. No one has ever said that about my name before. I don't even think it *is* that kind of name; come on, that's a sign!

It has actually been on my mind to have this two-year memoir printed out and book bound to give it to my family and friends eventually. After all I am an ordinary person of modest intellect (generously speaking!) with no formal religious background. If I could summon my core beliefs and find my way through the past two years it might be comforting for others. It could be rewarding for me to share these experiences.

The message to my children or anyone else is you must maintain your convictions that it can all be handled; most often we do rise to the challenges we are given. I've learned that no matter what I go through, I must be aware and thankful for the "good things" that happen all around. For me, this was helpful to finding the strength to get through what I have faced.

Basically, I am a negative person and it has not been easy to remember the appreciation of the "little things in life," which helps so much. It has been easier to learn to be grateful for the friendships, kindnesses and love that I have enjoyed.

I am more aware of than ever is that "faith" makes everything more bearable. It does not matter to what degree or where you find it. It could be faith in your family, a friend, a pet's love, a spiritual connection, a doctor, a treatment or something else. A passion for your work or a particular interest can also bring purpose and fulfillment. What is important is that *something* brings you strength and a little more peace.

In the beginning this journal was a way to remember exactly what was going on, how I made certain decisions, and especially how I handled my crisis. Of greater importance was actually how my relationships with others enabled me to cope well and move forward. Anyway, I am thinking about what I would like to do with my project when it is finished.

I have managed to talk to or text my friends. Ginny and I had a good visit one afternoon right after the memorial. She and Greg had a wedding in South Carolina and could not join us that day. I had not seen Colette, who was nursing a bad cold, since the memorial and we will get together soon.

Laura is very busy as always, but has been keeping in close touch. Art is having serious issues again and may need more treatments soon. We will be sending him only positive thoughts. We love them.

Our former neighbor stopped by last week while visiting her close friends across the street from us. She heard about Garry from our mutual friend Maryann and wanted to extend her condolences. Her boss's wife had ALS for five years. How awful! We are grateful that was not my brother's experience.

Baseball season has started again and though I haven't been quite as into that as of late, it is still a strong interest. The Yanks are doing OK, but pitching is their biggest problem—that's baseball. They are still fun to watch most days. This interest also gives Irwin and me lots to talk about. Mom is immediately bored by all sports chatter, which in itself strikes me with some humor. I am not sure why, but it does!

My plan is to keep journaling through Keith's graduation just a few weeks away. This is the most important, nicest, big event to happen to our immediate family for a long time. I cannot imagine rounding out these two years without including this day.

Well, who would have guessed this project would have seen me through so much? I realize now that my breast cancer journey will be ongoing. In the next few weeks I have three follow-up doctors' appointments. The estrogen blocker should be required for more than four more years. All the annual diagnostics and in-between appointments make me feel like this issue is very much with me; though it might be viewed as maintenance.

Easter was very nice. We all made contributions. It is really the only way to handle all that is required for a family bash. My sister-in-law's children and grandchildren joined our usual crew. This made it different and more fun. Since Barb's sister, daughter and daughter-in-law were on board with her I stepped away from getting involved with much of the cleanup work that I often do.

Her daughter-in-law had prophylactic breast surgery, meaning she chose to remove her breasts as a precaution before any cancer was found, based on family history. I was interested in talking with her in particular. Actually, we did not talk about our experiences in any detail. We simply acknowledged we were doing well and that we both try to maintain a positive attitude about our situations. She is a very strong young woman with four children and she seems to be handling things quite well. This made me very happy to see her.

We talked mostly about her being a dedicated special education teacher. As my dad, mom, step-father and brother were all involved in these programs in different ways I was very interested.

Everyone enjoyed the day. Anne and her boyfriend were absent as she was feeling sick. Later on, Keith went back to school to finish up his senior year at Rutgers.

I worked the next day at the nursing home. This was the first time I have worked since before Garry's passing. It was a bit strange. I had been back to see Alex, but this workday felt odd. When my break and lunch times came, I felt lost not rushing to visit my brother. That was what I did at every opportunity when I worked there before.

I actually tried to visit Alex but he was not available. I walked around just kind of reliving our experiences while Garry was there. It made me feel pretty peculiar and somewhat "blue." The people there were very nice, and most expressed condolences. I knew I would be back in a few days for a general memorial program to honor all residents who passed away in the last few months.

Mom and I attended the memorial at the nursing home. It was too impersonal regarding my brother and that left me unsettled. The Rabbi did his best to describe each person and included personal stories. Some of those remembered sounded like well-loved and admired additions to this home and others were much less familiar. My brother did have the distinction of being the youngest long-term resident. For me this was an unnecessary event. I imagine other people felt differently.

Later after dinner, we attended Cara's school Spring Concert. It was pleasant and a welcome change of pace for this day.

Thursday, April 29, I went into NY to see my oncologist with Anne. Apparently I am among a very small group who are pretty disinterested in the Prince William and Kate's nuptials this morning. Perhaps this was because I was anxious to speak with my doctor about some issues that might be related to my medication. I also was missing the impromptu tribute at Garry's work place today, which I felt very badly about.

When I got to the doctor's office I was asked to fill out a detailed form. I was careful to tick-off all the symptoms and conditions I wanted to bring to my doctor's attention this time.

My doctor came into the room to see me and to my surprise she had an extreme case of laryngitis. Her nurse was reading the scribbled notes from her pad to me, but the demeanor and general manner was uncomfortable and awkward. So, the visit was brief and less beneficial than I had hoped for. The good thing was I need not return for another three months.

It was silly of me not to voice my concerns, which will wait until next time. I just did not feel up to the effort. My usual bloodwork was taken and we were on our way home. Now, I am really upset that I missed my brother's work-place tribute to him. How sad.

MAKING PLANS
AND MOVING FORWARD

John contacted our mechanic about finding a good used car for Cara. He told John that his son's car would be perfect for her. This came relatively quickly to us. We decided it would be a better situation for Cara, than to use either of our mini-vans. We had not even told her we would consider buying her a car. So, she will be mighty surprised!

Anne had gotten a used car from her grandparents when she got her license. That helped us out a lot. Keith had gotten an old car from Uncle Leon when he first started driving. This was a huge deal as it saw him through college and he is still driving it. We make fun of the car because of its size and condition, but thank God for that old tank! When we told Cara about the car we bought her she couldn't believe it.

Our mechanic dropped the car off on Friday night. The mini-vans we drive were not working so well for this girl. If it wasn't such a well-cared-for used car we would not have considered the purchase.

Later that evening when she came home, I could hear Cara and a friend yelling in excitement on our driveway. Cara ran inside afterward still glowing with delight about her "beautiful car." We still had to register it and get new plates before she could drive it. She was already thrilled! Oh, when you make someone *this* happy, it's a special feeling. Let's hope it is a good move for a long time to come.

Saturday evening we went to dinner with my friend Marian and her husband, who we seldom see since our boys graduated high school together. Wow, both of the boys are graduating from college in a couple of weeks. How is this possible so soon? It was a relaxing early evening as is their custom. After an emotional and hectic week, this was needed. Marian and I are not great at keeping in touch; however, she is better at arranging these infrequent dates and it was good to keep up the friendship.

Sunday, as I was getting ready for bed I happened to turn on the TV. There was a "Special Report." The President would be making a statement after midnight. Reporters were speculating that he would announce the death of Osama bin Laden at the hands of our Special Forces. Wow, this was amazing news!

I'm more the appreciator of covert actions, I guess. This operation was necessary to ridding the world of this radical maniac. However, the idea that we had planned the execution of anyone and were willing to report it openly was nevertheless shocking for me to hear. I knew we were rightly hunting him down, but I imagined that he would be brought in and imprisoned if possible, first. This did not sound like that kind of mission. It all sounded a little perverse.

I am glad he is gone. Yet I am scared that this is the way of our world now. Not to be totally naïve, I get "assassination." I just thought we would find out what happened in a different way and time. Silly me. For days the story had slight variations and the same outcome. I hate to even dignify such a person on these pages. Unfortunately, it is very important news and must be noted.

It was May 2, which is also Keith's birthday. We will celebrate on his next visit home as he has to take exams now. He was OK about this, but seemed stressed by the pressure of graduation, which does concern me.

This week is about catching up with friends, and buckling down to take care of some things long on my "to-do list." I finally got a chance to sit and chat with Colette who was feeling better. Her mom was still heavily on her mind, but I felt she was calmer about her passing. She is excited for her daughter who is soon to leave on a college mission-trip for three weeks. As moms do, we support our children while we worry about the details.

Friday, John and I decided that we should make plans to have a family graduation party at a restaurant. We generally don't consider such expenses as something we can handle. Truthfully, I have wanted to plan a party for quite some time. We have never had real anniversary parties, even for our milestones. On John's fortieth birthday, I had a surprise house-party for him. Other than that, we have lots of the family hosting duties (holidays, family birthdays and BBQs) at our home. One occasion is much like the one before. After the challenges in the last two years, something special was needed.

This reminded me how my brother used to make every birthday an event to be celebrated. I would tell him that not each one was a big deal as we get older. He always replied, "Well, I think they are and I *want* to have a party." He always did.

Now, though we are still missing Garry very much, it is time to celebrate Keith's graduation. Summer parties are tough in our home, as our den air conditioner does very little to make a difference on a hot day. We didn't want to worry about the weather or the fuss. Therefore, I booked a party at a restaurant about ten minutes away. Maybe John and I will enjoy hosting more without the preparations and work in our home.

This will be a good way to thank our families for all they do to support us. The contract is signed and a buffet is on the books. I feel very frivolous!

Cara had to take her SAT test early Saturday morning. The rest of the day and weekend was about Mother's Day for the most part. We just had Mom and Irwin, who had breakfast with Vicki and Paul before they went into NY to see Jen. John's Aunt Betty, Cara, Anne and Dave were also here. We did not include anyone else, as we will see them all on June 18, at our party. The day was quiet and very manageable.

It allowed us some extra time with Aunt Betty who is planning to sell her home and move to Ohio soon to be near one of her daughters. She and I have a special relationship and I will miss her very much.

My family gifted me with a new cell phone. I had the same old phone for seven years and it needed to be replaced. Anne set it up for me, and I was feeling pleased with the addition of a keyboard and picture capacity. As usual I am not even running a slow race to being a techno-savvy person. I am happy with my simple, no-Internet capacity new phone.

Still working hard to finish school, Keith admittedly was struggling to complete the heavy load he brought on himself in the end. His first few years were perhaps too focused on football and rugby interests. It finally caught up with him as he raced to make it to the goal line. We had told him from the start, "This is a four-year program." He managed to finalize his studies with the addition of only a couple of summer classes last year. In the end, he made sure he was a May 2011 Graduate. Good job, son!

Keith came home for a day. It allowed him to chill out and to assure us everything was on track. His cap and gown were picked up and ready. There seemed to be an air of disbelief and a surreal feeling about the upcoming event. We were all looking forward to seeing the ceremony on Sunday.

Meanwhile, I had another big day in the city, having scheduled two doctor appointments on Thursday, May 12. Again Anne drove me in. First, we went to my plastic surgeon. It was the yearly checkup and he was as always aloof and confident. He liked what he saw and told me to return in a year. Then, I told him I was having some general itching problems, which I wanted to be sure was not an allergy reaction to the implants. I was also suspicious that this condition might be caused by the estrogen blocker. He quickly dismissed all my concerns by commenting, "This is definitely not an allergic reaction to the implants." The plastic surgeon said that I should see my local dermatologist and made his usual quick escape.

Anne and I stopped to have breakfast as our next appointment at the breast surgeon was not until 2:00. After eating I called the breast surgeons' office to see if we could see her earlier; expecting that cancelations had occurred since they left a message on my phone saying my doctor was not in today and appointments were being covered by someone else. That worked well and the routine exam was moved up to 12:30.

The covering doctor was very cordial and talkative. I told her about my concerns and we spoke for a while. She agreed with my oncologist's office which had given me some telephone advice earlier in the week. This young practitioner seemed very interested, and assured me that I seemed well despite my complaints. My next appointment with my breast surgeon is also for one year from now. This was also good news.

My next plan was to go home and cook a meal for Laura to take home to her family tomorrow after our visit. I made them an Italian pot roast which is usually a winner. The portion was large so that they can freeze some for another day. I hope that this little gesture will provide a welcome treat for them. I want to help my friends and I recall how great these considerations were for us. Laura and I don't see each other much now. Art's therapy is tougher this time; she needs to spend more time supporting him. I completely understand. It breaks my heart to know about the struggle that they are now facing. We are praying for them.

After a nice visit, Laura took home the dinner I had told her to expect to have today. I included a marble cheese cake to make the treat complete. She and I share a serious sweet-tooth and I knew this would go over well. It felt good to do something for these special friends.

Keith came home Friday night before the big event. He took Cara driving the next morning—what a good big brother. Then, he left us and we knew the next time we saw each other would be in the midst of the commotion of graduation day.

Saturday afternoon Mom's friends Joan and Marvin drove from Pennsylvania for a visit. They had made a DVD of an old family vacation we shared as young families together. It captured my Dad and brother and their youngest son, who had passed away years ago, also. It was a quick time capsule of one vacation. Marvin was not a careful cameraman, as he rapidly panned across each scene quickly. Even so, it was a lovely opportunity to remember old times, and the friendship that has endured time and significant losses. We love to see Joan and Marvin, who are like family in our hearts. It was a great visit and we promised to visit them this summer. Mom was very happy to see her friends again.

Tomorrow, we will get up very early to leave by 7:15 for the mornings' general Rutgers Graduation Ceremony in the football stadium.

My Mom, Irwin, Mary, Bob, Anne and Dave are also planning to attend. However, weather reports are calling for heavy rain and storms. We were keeping our fingers crossed on this turning out better than the forecasted predictions. The main problem is that there is a second smaller ceremony at the Communications Sciences School at 6:00 in the evening. The day will be complicated enough without bad weather included.

Cara came home from seeing another high school play. She was determined to bang out her review for submission. This was fairly easy as she excels in writing. She had to e-mail the review before going to sleep; our morning's schedule was too tight to include remembering to do that before we left. I admired her proficiency and determination. With a touch of a key her piece was finished and sent off.

We were all tired and knew a little sleep before the main event was wise. Everyone was becoming anxious. I was worrying about Keith, and whether he would be on time and where he was supposed to be tomorrow. Then I thought, *He made it this far on his own—so tomorrow should be easy!*

GRADUATION

Sunday morning, May 15, 2011, the rain was so heavy that we couldn't decide if anyone should go ahead to the ceremony outdoors. Of course, we felt that John, Cara and I had to go no matter what the weather brought.

Mom and Irwin were outside at 7:00 and it was pouring so heavily, they could not get out of their car. We were waiting for the right moment to run outside. Mary phoned to say they would come to the later ceremony, and offered to drive Mom and Irwin with them. We all agreed this was a better plan.

As soon as the rain lightened up a bit, we ran into our car and were off to the first ceremony. We arrived and parked far from the stadium. Then, we took the shuttle bus provided for this occasion. We found our way to the bleachers and sat in a light, on-and-off-again rain. Rain ponchos were handed out which helped from blocking other people with umbrellas. It was a bit hot and sticky under the plastic but tolerable.

We watched as the stadium floor filled with graduates. This became an endless red and black stream. Even though they started the actual ceremony quite late to accommodate the graduates' arrivals, more people just kept coming on the field up until the ceremony's end.

The Rutgers' band and Glee Club were wonderfully talented and enjoyable. The event had the usual "Pomp and Circumstance" and was quite extraordinary in size alone. There were officially over eleven thousand graduates this year, and I believe the ceremony was attended by over six thousand of them in the morning.

The guest speaker was Toni Morrison, author and Nobel Prize winner. She did not paint the most flattering picture of our world today. She challenged these young men and woman to make the transformations needed to put things on a more positive track. She told them, "Do not to look for happiness in your future, look for meaningfulness in your future." It was not all together optimistic or upbeat as speeches go. It was thought-provoking and interesting. I wondered if it might be viewed as being a bit too dismal for this crowd.

John remembered his alma mater's song and sang along to it, ". . . along the banks of the old Raritan . . ." Oh my! It was fantastic to see the event, though we had no clue where our son was. Keith found us at the completion of the festivities.

It was hot and muggy, and we all needed something to eat and drink. When I say, "we," I mean *everybody* there. That's when things got crazy. Huge numbers of people were anxious to leave the stadium to get to different places. Some had earlier second ceremonies than we did. Other people had reservations at restaurants nearby to get to. Wherever they were off to, they were all desperate to leave the grounds. Most needed to catch a shuttle bus back to their cars.

This was the first time I ever felt what it was like to be caught in a mob. We were pushed and shoved. It was mighty uncomfortable for the one-and-a-half hours that we tried to leave that area. I was relieved that Grandma and Grandpa were not in this crowd! They have definitely regained their usual and admirable vitality, but they would not have enjoyed this part of the festivities. The police were basically more of a hindrance than a help. At last, we got on the bus and were on our way to our car.

Keith suggested a restaurant nearer to where he works. That got us away from the crowds in the local places near the university. We found a quiet restaurant that Keith appeared never to have actually gone to before. The waitresses had short-shorts, mid-drift blouses and belly piercings. The names of food selections and sayings on the walls were all very "guy" oriented. The men's restroom door had a silhouette of a pair of boxer-shorts while the women's restroom door had one of a thong. We were mostly glad to find a quiet place to sit and grab a bite. Already tired and starving, this worked out fine, although it was a bit of a man-cave.

We called Anne and Mary and suggested that they not plan to eat down near the college later. We knew we couldn't wait for them to arrive, as we were starved. It was unlikely that they could easily find a decent place in time and make it to the second venue.

Mary and Bob brought Mom and Irwin down. Bob chose to sightsee around the campus and got lost in the process. They did finally make it with time to spare. Anne and Dave were also in the area. They unwisely tried to stop to eat close to the college on their way. That proved to be a bad move, as my prediction of difficulty was correct.

Finally, we all met up and sat together to see the second indoor ceremony. We were glad we had made it this far. This time, we could actually see Keith come in and sit in his row and go up for his diploma (not the real diploma which is mailed home later).

The Rutgers' football player who was paralyzed in a game injury earlier this year was in attendance. He received a standing ovation for his inspiring courage, recovery and attendance on this day. You could feel all the prayers and good wishes going out to him; it was an intense and emotional moment.

The ceremony continued. With the second event it felt more official—Keith had done it! Yay! Afterward, we stepped outside and took some photos. We talked with Keith and his friends. As is his custom, Keith was not letting us in on what he wanted to do. Eventually, we decided to let him go off with a friend to work out their evening.

We were exhausted and ready to go home. It was a special day that was typically poorly planned on our part. The bad weather had proven to be an obstacle by making things a little crazier. Still, it was all great—you go, Keith!

There is one funny note: I had a graduation card for our son with a long personal message for him I wrote before the ceremony. Besides expressing our pride in him, I spoke confidently about our hopes for a very bright future. I emphasized wanting him to *"find happiness."* Hey, I am his mother and not the guest speaker!

Graduation is over. We have the party planned for next month. I am hoping most everyone will be able to join us for a little celebrating. It was my intention to end this journal with the graduation event. However, I believe now it will end with the family party.

I think this celebration is very important for us all. For Keith it is a well-noted milestone among his greatest fans. For John and me it is that, too. Also it is an acknowledgement of *our* accomplishment in seeing him through this achievement. We want to thank our entire family for their unending support. In addition, it is a way of saying: We've been through a lot of serious problems; yet, let's enjoy sharing the good times we can together. I know Garry would agree.

OPPORTUNITIES

Things have settled down again now that graduation has taken place. My undiagnosed general itching is an annoyance. This seems to be like the situation I experienced last summer after the bug bite infection on my leg. Then, my GP thought I was not coping well and needed to find ways to de-stress. I did not agree, but I had not pursued the issue either.

I have had conversations with the oncologist office regarding various issues. Some of my symptoms and complaints are common among women who have gone through similar breast cancer treatments. They suggested a simple routine for me and advised that I increase my fluids daily.

Unfortunately the dermatology appointment could not be made for three weeks from my initial call. My condition became more aggravated, and I ended up at my GP for a consult. A new doctor diagnosed me with a virus; she agreed that I should also see the dermatologist the next week.

Meanwhile, Cara lucked into a summer job starting next month. Cara will be an assistant exercise coach in pre-school classes. This is great and makes her one of the lucky kids who actually has a summer job. Cara is delighted at the prospect of having some money to spend—I mean save, right? The gas money will definitely come in handy.

Cara and I decided she needed to shop for new sandals. We ran to the mall after school and found two pairs we liked. We continued to look around and also found a black print casual dress. I said, "It's very Lea Michelle." She understood I was referring to *GLEE* and Cara accepted the compliment. I was thinking, *Wonderful dress for the graduation party.* The day's successes made us both happy.

Keith came home with the intention of having a couple of free meals, getting some laundry assistance, and giving me a hand with a trip for water, the last being a great help for me. He was excited about a job interview he had recently. While we were out he was informed via his cell phone e-mail that the company was "not ready to make a decision." It is not easy to explain to anyone who thinks their interview went very well, that maybe they are jumping ahead of themselves. John and I tried to lend some support.

My sister-in-law Rita called and asked for a favor. She was in need of help picking up her son Dan from college on Sunday. She was working and her other children were not around to help her out. John was happy to pick up his nephew. He had a lot less to move out than we were used to with Keith at the end of the school year. John made the trip and was gone for most of the afternoon. He enjoyed helping his nephew and his sister out. We were glad she called.

One thing that I have learned is: When someone tells you *how* you can help them specifically, it is a "gift" they give to you. We try to be thoughtful in our efforts, but often we don't know what is most needed. It makes you feel great to actually do something meaningful. Knowing that someone trusts they can ask you for help is a huge compliment. Hey, sometimes you cannot meet every request and need, but you do your best.

This time on Sunday convinced me to do something that I had been thinking about. Last month, I saw an article about meeting a couple who has written a new book at a local book store. This interested me, as their book tells how to get your book published. This would be helpful to my idea of publishing my journal. When John had gotten this last-minute plan for the afternoon, I felt I had no excuse not to go. The established authors, Arielle Eckstut and David Henry Sterry, were entertaining and informative. I just stood taking it all in and found it fascinating. In this small local store, were other people like me; we were dreaming of writing something worthwhile to share.

I saw someone I recognized and spoke to him afterward. We spoke about a number of topics before wishing each other luck with our books. My head was spinning. I left with a signed book in hand.

—✸—

My health problems were not resolving themselves and were becoming a real nuisance. Not only was I generally itchy, but I was aware of excessive hot flashes. Any temperature variation brought on more severe burning and itching. This meant even perspiration caused me great discomfort. What the heck?

Finally, I saw the dermatologist and this appointment brought no answers either. As I had been put on a medication by my GP, which needed more time, there was nothing this doctor could do. This doctor found two areas on my skin to biopsy anyway. She explained that there is a link between breast cancer and increased skin melanomas. Great, more worries ahead.

LOTS OF CHANGES

This is the week the *Oprah* shows ends. Her twenty-five year reign is ending with much anticipation. I am looking forward to seeing these last few hour-long shows. I have watched her over many of these years.

I admire Oprah's accomplishments and dedication to helping others aspire to improve and change in positive ways. Her philanthropy is amazing and commendable. She is passionate about the power of the human spirit and education; she is a force. Mostly, I mention this as I have made quite a few references to her already.

Wednesday, May 25, on her last show Oprah stood alone and shared her experiences and insights. My thought was maybe this should have been Monday's program. The two-hour surprise extravaganzas could have followed. Well, I don't imagine Oprah needs *my* advice to continue her success. Listen, I am kind of disappointed that she will not be plugging my book someday!

So, *Oprah's* gone, but my itch is not. I went to my gynecologist to see if he thought some of my concerns were typically due to changes since the oophorectomy and amount of estrogen in my body. This doctor sees women who have gone through similar adjustments and I trust him. I had not seen him since my original diagnosis. He was the doctor who had called a number of times just to check up on how I was doing. That is rare these days among the medical profession and I have an enormous respect for him. He assured me that I appeared to have all the "normal" signs, but he performed some routine tests to be sure there were no overlooked infections.

My gynecologist was fussing with a new computer program while he entered information about me while we spoke together. I told him that *I* was not a computer person. He was surprised that I was not taking advantage of this marvelous resource and suggested that I should use the Internet. I left thanking him for his help. He will let me know if anything shows up from the tests.

I told John about my visit and then he decided to do some computer diagnosis investigation of his own. John called me in to read information regarding a "systemic yeast infection." I recognized many facts and symptoms that paralleled my situation perfectly. We were convinced we had the answer. The one thing that concerning us was, "this could be fatal."

The next day, I called my oncologist. She listened and seemed puzzled, too. She asked me to continue with my doctors regarding these problems and concerns. She also thought that I should take a three-week break from the blocker at this time.

Later the GP called suggesting more bloodwork in hopes of finding a clue as to what was going on. This was getting ridiculous and very frustrating.

While going from one doctor's conversation to another, I received a text from Laura. Her husband was feeling better today and she was so happy. I knew this felt like a real breakthrough and I was relieved for them both. We *all* really take our health for granted too much of the time.

Keith came home and mentioned he was desperate for new sneakers. We went shopping to solve that problem. We had no difficulty and in short time managed to make a selection that satisfied his requirements. Sneakers are always one of his favorite purchases.

The rest of his weekend was going to be busy. Keith must move out of his old apartment and then, move into his new place in one or two days. He is sharing a house with a number of boys down the street from where he is now. Keith is employed at the same job he started at last summer, and where he worked part-time through the last year of school. This apartment is close to his job. It does allow him to live away from home and I understand the attractiveness in that. Now that he has graduated from college, Keith is wasting no time and already is looking for a new job.

Using John's van Keith made a number of trips back and forth with his belongings during the next several days. Many of his things were left in our living room for a few days. Keith was working, so he was quite busy. When I noticed some unfamiliar and pungent odors coming from the laundry in my living room, I decided to pitch in and do some of his laundry.

First, I managed to take all his bedding straight to the laundromat in town. John had Keith's car, which they had traded with one another, and left it to be serviced. We knew Keith had been unable to find the time for this maintenance. What a lucky guy; Mom and Dad really had his back!

By the end of the day, we felt good knowing certain things were in better shape.

Memorial weekend was quiet for us. Knowing Keith would be with us Saturday I cooked a big stew. At the last minute, I invited Mary and Bob to join us for supper. We had not seen them since Keith's Graduation ceremony. They came by and we had an early evening together. We were planning to host our party in a couple of weeks and were not particularly interested in doing the BBQ duties on the holiday this time. Frankly, we were pooped! The kids were all pretty busy with their weekend activities and did not care much.

Monday was Memorial Day and Vicki's birthday. She, Paul and Jennifer were planning a city day. However, my sister insisted on taking all of us out for breakfast at the diner. Keith was too busy moving; and Anne's boyfriend did not feel well, so they were both absent. The rest of us met up for a very casual and easy meal. We were glad to share a bit of Vicki's birthday and this was her way of hosting the holiday. I gave her a coffee shop gift card knowing how much she loves that!

Now, I haven't mentioned my Yankees much. That is because it has been up and down with them. They are struggling more than not. The pitching staff has been riddled with injuries and problems. They do have C.C. Sabathia and incomparable Mo, Mariano Rivera; so, anything is still possible. I am savoring what I believe is my favorite player's, Jorge Posada, last season. I am partial to catchers, who I feel have the hardest job on the team. Keith, of course, was a catcher when he played baseball when he was younger. The baseball season still occupies much of our relaxation time. Go, Yanks!

Tuesday, Colette and I got together for a couple of hours. We laughed over many silly things that came up and it was especially fun to see her today. When I told her I had to run to my hair appointment, she frowned at the idea of me going too short again. I love short hair.

I left my friend and went to meet my fate. It turned out to be the best cut I have gotten in years. I came away feeling like a "new and improved" woman—just what I needed! Short, but not too short. It's sassy and manageable. I love it! By the time I see my friend again, my hair might be long enough to satisfy her, but probably not.

The next day I went to my GP and we did more bloodwork. She will let me know about the results next week.

RISING STARS AND MORE

The weekend came and we were looking forward to the critics' awards program on Sunday evening. This is a high school version of the Tony Awards. Cara was nominated for Best Comedic Actress in a Musical and for Best Junior CAPPI (11th grade critic). This was exciting and we knew it meant a lot to her. Several other students from our school were nominated in different categories.

Keith came home on Saturday afternoon. He, John and I had dinner together as Cara was out with her buddies. I nagged Keith about getting a lock on his bedroom door in his new apartment and he rudely answered back to me. I got annoyed at being treated in this manner. We were all tired and irritable. John tried to make attempts at calming the situation down and soon decided to abandon us both by taking a nap.

After a cool-down period, I spoke with my son. I told him that I had made sure he had gotten lots of help all week long, and *that* alone should have entitled me better treatment. Yes, Keith is a great son, who is helpful in many ways. We love him and yes, I worry about him. His former apartment nearby was burglarized, and so I felt justified in my concern.

Keith saw me getting upset and insisted on me sitting down to have a real talk with him. It enabled him to get lots of things off his chest. He hides more about his feelings than I ever realized. We talked for hours and I tried to listen carefully. I think with all that has been going on in the last couple of years here, Keith has felt as though he needed to keep some things even more bottled up.

I also think that post-graduation is a very odd time for many people. Wow, it is over! Now, what's next? Keith is working, but simultaneously looking for a better opportunity. It is a time for big adjustments. *Not* to be a student all of a sudden is one of those changes that can throw you off. I was pretty sure this was all "normal stuff" going on with him.

Actually, I am pleased we got to have this long and informative talk together. I think we both felt better afterward. It is unnecessary to detail more about our conversation. Just the way he expressed himself makes me feel better; I am very proud of Keith. I will try to be more supportive in other ways than is usual for me. He *still* cannot be disrespectful and he will try to be more careful, also. We all make mistakes.

Sunday, we could all feel Cara's excitement and nervousness. Keith decided to stay later than he had planned to see the ceremony. He took Cara out for a driving lesson earlier and they both seemed pleased with her progress.

Anne and Dave were helping Grandma and Grandpa with their garage sale all day. Anne thought some of Garry's Coke collectibles were valuable and knew she could look up all the information on the Internet on her cell phone. Mom and Irwin were very impressed with the technology and people-skills the kids had. Mostly, they really enjoyed the interest and time that Anne and Dave showed them. It was unsolicited and hugely appreciated. Though the day did not prove lucrative, they had fun. It was a long day for them. They all wished Cara well, but decided to wait and hear about the results later from us.

Cara had to be at school all afternoon to rehearse the opening number and help set up. We arrived on time. It was fun to see bits of the other plays performed on our stage or shown on tape. This branch organization is made up of a small group of high schools, yet it is impressive to find so much talent among them. The productions were all ambitious and professional-like.

Our school came away with several awards. Cara got the "Best Comedic Actress in a Musical" and we were thrilled for her. She was just bursting with joy and accomplishment! I might have controlled myself a little more, as I yelled my head off in support and with great pride! John and Keith were quieter and at the same time hardily enjoying the moment.

We called Anne and Grandma separately and they were very happy to get the news. I couldn't believe how exciting it was!

Monday, I called Ginny for a walk. It was great to see her and get in some exercise again. I really miss doing both on a consistent basis. The heat and my itch are a poor combination, yet I must try to get back to this.

Laura and I decided that we would get together on Thursday. Her birthday was last Saturday. I went to a store with Cara that sells accessories and found a funky necklace for my friend. My mom had given me a Coca-Cola tin from Garry's collection for Laura, and a T-shirt from the charity walk sponsored by his workplace. They had "WE LOVE Garry B." added on the sleeve in memory of him.

I am looking forward to seeing Laura. I missed our visits terribly. It was difficult to see Garry together as his ALS progressed; at the same time, it brought us all a little closer.

My GP called to report the bloodwork was all fine. She suggested that I take some over-the-counter allergy pills once a day along with two antacid tablets for two weeks. If I improve then perhaps an appointment with an allergist is in order. I will try this and maybe it can provide some relief.

The weather has been really oppressive the last couple of days. Mostly, I have taken advantage by working on my journal instead of running around.

My gynecologist called to make sure I received the results that all my tests came back fine. We spoke and I told him that John and I had read some information about systemic yeast infections. I told him that many of the symptoms matched mine and we thought this might offer some explanation regarding my itch and other complaints. He paused and asked, "Do you think you're a very sick person? Why would you look up something like that?"

I reminded him about the computer conversation in his office and explained John's finding the information. This was his response: "I meant that you should learn about things like how Venice was built, or something else that you're interested in. I never meant for you to self-diagnose!" My response was, "Well, my itch is what I'm interested in! I don't care about Venice!" He laughed and reassured me that we were way off.

The week was filled with more of the usual day to day tasks. I was looking forward to spending time with Laura and assembled her gift. I put the t-shirt from the annual fundraising walk inside the Coca-Cola tin as a remembrance for Laura to have. She also appeared to like the necklace Cara and I picked out for her. Typically Laura was gracious showing her enjoyment over this little fuss.

She and I were anxious to go out to have our traditional birthday lunch. We decided on a Mexican restaurant we both like. It was just-the-ticket to a delicious meal and a couple of relaxing hours. Laura and I talked a great deal more about our children. There are always family stories to share. These provided us with many laughs. She also mentioned that her husband's chemo treatments are harsher this time and that was weighing on them both.

I called John's Aunt Betty today forgetting that her grandson and his girlfriend were visiting from Ohio. I sent them a card after I learned of his girlfriend's breast cancer diagnosis as I felt compelled to offer a little encouragement. I was reminded how touched I was by the unexpected sources of extended kindnesses. Val and I had only met once almost five years ago. Aunt Betty gave her the phone so that we could speak together. She seemed like a very sweet gal with a good head on her shoulders. We quickly traded all kinds of detailed information and facts.

I expect her experience will be different in many ways from my own. It was interesting to speak with her and I was pleased to make this quick connection. Hopefully, she found some comfort in my interest. Val will be added to my thoughts.

PARTY TIME

The focus of the next week and couple of days was about getting ready for Keith's graduation party. Also, the day after that is Father's Day. Oops, almost forgot about that one. Guess there is some shopping to do.

I diligently purchased all that we needed to pull our simple little family celebration off. First, I found an understated summer dress. I wanted to look like the hostess of an informal Saturday luncheon party and this selection fit the bill.

The largest project was making the center pieces for the four guest tables and various other decorations required to transform the room where we were having the event. It did not seem necessary to go the flowers route as Keith just isn't that kind of guy.

My idea was to have large beer mugs filled with chocolate candies, wrapped in the red and black school colors as center pieces. Then I found little red graduation tassels to hang from the handles with black curled ribbon bows, which I would make. In addition, there would be three red and black graduation balloons tied to each handle. After stopping at about eight different stores I finally ended up with all the supplies needed to accomplish my envisioned pieces. When I assembled one, it became clear to me that I had to have a matt, or cloth to sit the mug on to complete the proportion and desired effect. It had to be black, and my task continued.

These pieces would be assembled at the restaurant on the morning of the party. I made the curled ribbon bows with the tassels hanging on them in the center in advance. This turned out to be good planning on my part as they were time consuming. Along my travels, I found other graduation motif items to splash around the party room and it seemed we were prepared enough.

Shopping was not completed until Father's Day was also taken care of. Grandpa was easy. I found an exceptionally nice-looking, medium-weight Yankee jacket. Irwin is such a big fan and a snazzy dresser that I was sure this was a winner.

John was tougher to shop for. I had no idea what to get him. He finally asked for a couple of new dress shirts and ties to freshen up his work wardrobe. The children wanted in on whatever I could find, as they were also out of ideas this time. After quite a bit of effort and consideration I found everything for our group gift. I like to shop, but this was all a little much even for me. Finally, I felt we were ready.

Now, I was even more appreciative that I was not cleaning my home and preparing food all week in addition to all these errands. It was important for us to have a manageable celebration. We all needed a wonderful and hopeful occasion to share. Holding the party in a restaurant meant much less work. It especially meant John and I could have more fun. Still, at this point, I was nervous and worrying about details and arrangements. I had decided that this should remain an intimate family event. It would not include even our few close friends. I didn't want to insult anyone; it simply felt most right to have this small family celebration.

One distraction and break to my party efforts came on Friday when I met Colette for coffee. We agreed to a short meeting nearby; this is tough for us to stick to and in the end, we spent a quick couple of hours together. It was a good way to slow down a bit. We promised to talk again after the party next week.

Laura was away with a couple of our high school classmates she remains close with. I am happy for this mini-vacation my friend deserves. Actually she had been away with these same friends the day of my mastectomy almost two years ago. Since Laura's youngest son graduates from high school on Wednesday, she will have to cut this time away short. She texted to wish me well on our party; we will talk again after her son's graduation.

Saturday, June 18, came. Cara had offered to help me set up the party decorations at about 11:00. We went to the restaurant with all the items to be assembled and placed around the room. After a good hour of work we had placed everything exactly as we wanted. It looked great. Then we went home and quickly dressed.

Keith had arrived home while we were gone and appeared relatively unconcerned about the event. We arrived at the restaurant before 1:30 and Keith seemed impressed as he saw the room for the first time. About ten minutes later our guests started to arrive.

Mom and Irwin picked up John's Aunt Betty and brought her to the party. She will be moving in a few weeks to live close by to her daughter. It is heartbreaking for her to leave the home she has enjoyed for well over sixty years. This gathering is a perfect opportunity for her to see all the members of John's and my families that she would want to see before moving. Mom, Irwin and I intend to take her out for breakfast before she leaves. This also made seeing her today easier for me. We are enormously fond of one another.

Unfortunately, several people we had hoped to share the day with couldn't attend. We missed them knowing it becomes almost impossible to make a date work for everyone. We were twenty-four people at our final count.

All our guests arrived on time and in good humor. John and I have been fortunate that our families have always mixed and enjoyed each other's company throughout the years. We spent the better part of four hours sharing this special occasion together. The food was delicious and the room very private and comfortable.

Keith was a low-key, cool "guest of honor." It was obvious to me that he was delighted with his party. The cousins; Mary Kate, Dan, Rob, Keith, Cara, Anne and Anne's boyfriend Dave had a great time together.

Mom, Irwin, my Aunt Betty and John's Aunt Betty seemed equally thrilled to be with us. Those four are quite an inspiration, really! Vicki, Paul, Mary, Bob, Tom, Barbara and Rita were ready to party. My cousins Peter, Carol, Eric and his girlfriend Robin were in good spirits, too. We were so glad they all made the trip to celebrate with us. Everyone had a wonderful time casually mingling throughout the afternoon.

John prepared a moderately short speech about Keith. It was sweet, flattering, heartfelt and a bit humorous. I believe he cut it shorter then intended when he became slightly and uncharacteristically emotional. His speech meant a lot to Keith who likewise tries not to display this side often.

Shortly afterward I told a couple of quick stories about Keith, poking fun mostly at him and maybe a little at John and myself. We felt great about treating our entire family today and having expressed our pride in our son's tremendous accomplishment.

Keith was happy with the party, the fuss and the recognition. He thanked us many times before he left to go back to his new apartment on Sunday night. This celebration will always be a wonderful memory.

Sunday morning Vicki and Paul arranged for Mom and Irwin, along with our family of five, plus Dave to meet for a Father's Day breakfast at the diner. It was not easy to get ready for the early meal, as I did not sleep well Saturday night. The couple of cups of coffee and chocolates I ate at the party really hit me. So, with about an hour of sleep we joined this additional family treat. We were all pleased about the party yesterday. Yay!

Vicki and Paul planned to go in to the city later to meet up with Jennifer and a couple of friends. Mom and Irwin were off to spend a quiet afternoon with Alex at the nursing home. They knew his daughters were at a family wedding and he would be alone. It was a beautiful day; Alex would definitely want to sit outside to enjoy the weather.

We went home and Anne and Dave came back with us to give John his cards and gifts. It became impossible for me to keep my eyes from closing. This was so not like me. After a short time, I excused myself to the den and fell off to sleep. Wow! I was shot, but in a good way. Much to my surprise I awakened three hours later.

John, Keith, Anne, Dave and Uncle Bob were off to hit some balls at the golf range together. Cara was busy working at the computer. I sat down to work on my journal, creating more permanence to our successful weekend and family event. I was thrilled about the weekend.

Reaching My Destination

Recognizing that I could be strong seemed to make me stronger. That is my experience. In the beginning of my journey it occurred to me that breast cancer wasn't the only thing that could kill me. The decisions I made were big and life-changing. What I can be certain of now is that I did not curl up in a ball, I did not sit around crying, and I never complained or asked, "Why me?" I knew I would find a way to do whatever had to be done. Did I make every right choice? I don't know. I made the right choices for me. They were not easy or nearly perfect ones.

My biggest goal was to show my children how to face something very difficult and still move forward in life. In the past two years, I have repeated this idea a number of times and in different ways; sometimes, even surprising me. *Facing the changes that come along is really what life is about.*

I needed to put my crisis in perspective. The balance that life provides for us became a little clearer in black and white. Sometimes terrible and unacceptable things do happen to us or those we love. In my case, writing has helped me remember how I handled everything; what was going on at this same time, and all the people I am indebted to for making both Garry's and my experiences easier to bear.

About my dear friends Laura, Ginny and Colette in particular, I must say that they have become closer to me and more treasured in these past two years.

If Yankee sports commentator and TV host of *Center Stage,* Michael Kay ever asked me, "Who would you want to be stuck in a fox hole with?" The choice would be difficult, but my answer would be, "Vicki." No one has more faith and positive-determination when it really counts! She is my sister and also my friend.

Of my extended family I can say that everyone helped so much. Some in ways that I may not have given credit to for their particular contributions; I know they forgive me. All their efforts and gestures have been greatly appreciated and not taken for granted. They are the best.

In regards to my immediate family, who are all remarkable and make any struggle worthwhile, I adore them. My daughter Anne was extraordinarily helpful; she was not chosen for "the fox hole" because

Anne is *always* late for everything. She has been wonderful. Keith and Cara could be counted on for their help; especially for keeping focused on all the important "normal" events in their lives, which was extremely important to me.

My husband John, who took on another extra-huge load, has been amazing. Just being my "better half" is difficult enough in a good year. I know it was even more so these past two years. It is also his generosity and understanding that has allowed me the time that writing this book has encompassed. *Not* choosing my husband for the "fox hole" isn't a reflection of my love for him; it does acknowledge my fear that our combined negativity might present a larger obstacle.

Mom and Irwin, who we all count on to share our strife and joys, are incredible. Facing this or any other crisis would be much more difficult without them.

Remembering my brother Garry, who taught us what real dignity and grace is, and built a life out of being a kind, loyal and loving person—he inspires and encourages me every time I think of him.

The remarkable acts of so many people have touched me. I will never forget Garry's friend who visited every Sunday morning for nine months leaving her two young children and husband to "hold down the fort" in her absence. Often, I think of the nursing homes' activity person who tried week after week to bring Garry some joy through her piano music. I will think of her whenever I hear the song *Take Me Out to the Ballgame*, which she always dedicated to my brother. There was my neighbor who gave me each at-home injection. I could go on, but I won't.

Remembered will be those people who spent difficult times with Garry and my family, and whose gestures have made a lasting impression. Appreciating kindnesses from those around me, and receiving the love of those dear to me, were powerful comforts through this challenging time. Not having to face these alone was an enormous and wonderful blessing.

Having been the recipient of so much support has shown me how sweet this life can be and made me stronger in the process. I found that helping others or receiving their help is deeply gratifying. We are not perfect, but sometimes we get closer. I did not decide to share this story because I thought it was so terribly unusual. I believe it is a good example how our trials and tribulations are special opportunities to strengthen connections to those around us. Of course, this is not meant as any justification for such things happening.

Certainly, there are never any guarantees that everything will work out as we want them to. Thank goodness many good things can happen while we are dealing with overwhelming problems. *That* is what helped me to keep going. Many of these experiences are what I really want to remember.

My son's college graduation feels like the right place to end. Fortunately, we all recognized the importance of not missing the opportunity to enjoy this significant milestone. Despite still deeply feeling my brother's loss and many of us dealing with other substantial issues, we had a great sense that this was valuable time to be shared together.

It was almost exactly two years ago, June 2009, when I found out that I had breast cancer. I realize now that my journey is still in its beginning. My hope is that like my sister, someday, I will boast of being a twenty-five year breast cancer survivor.

Life often surprises, usually challenges, and sometimes rewards us in many ways. At very least this makes our journeys interesting. There are certainly many hazards and delays along the way. For people like myself with a poor sense of direction there is always help. Having breast cancer is a big bump on my road. Garry would probably say, "Two big bumps!" I intend to continue ahead slowly and as safely as possible.

Here is my best advice to anyone faced with a difficult decision: Make the necessary changes in your direction whenever you *must* along your road. Accept the reality that sometimes the best plans need adjustments and alterations. You are not forever lost; there is usually another way to get to where you need to go. Ah, wait just a moment for that comforting word, "recalculating." This is life.

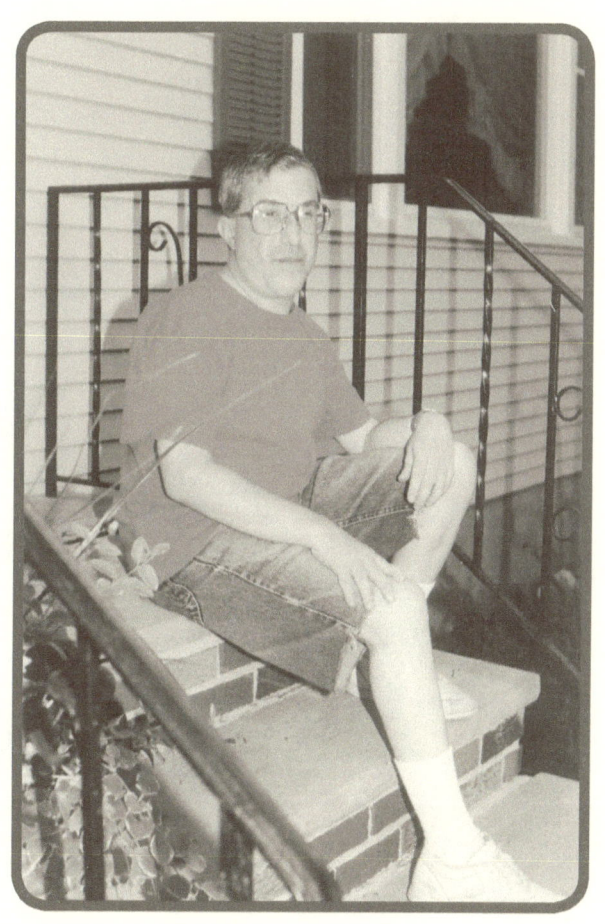

Garry Burros, 1955-2011

Acknowledgements

Upon the completion of my journal I began the task of deciding whether to offer my story to the public. A handful of people read the manuscript and offered feedback. I was gratified that each one found many worthwhile aspects of the book even in its' roughest form. To all my initial readers whose support both motivated and encouraged me, thank you!

A number of professionals, each of whom I almost stumbled upon, were instrumental in my pursuit to publish this book. I met editors, agents and writers who all read my manuscript and offered invaluable advice. They were extremely generous and enthusiastic. I listened to and learned from all of them.

In particular, I was extremely fortunate to make the acquaintance of Ann Bayer, a wonderful writer, and a mentor who allowed me to send her my book. After reading it in its original state, she munificently spent many, many hours teaching me how to sift through what I had written and clean it up. More importantly, she offered key pointers on writing that ultimately helped me to define my voice, enhancing the manuscript enormously! Her interest and friendship has been an unexpected bonus. Ann introduced me to *The Elements of Style* by William Strunk Jr. and E.B. White. This short book is a must for every writer and aspiring writer.

I would also like to extend my appreciation to Chris E., a writer and an editor who made several important suggestions at just the right time. His insights helped improve the telling of this complex story. He did this with a good nature and not for personal gain. Similarly, thanks to Gen W. for her assistance on the "perfect" book cover designed by Jen Gaily.

Last but not least, I am indebted to my family and friends who have shared these experiences with me and have graciously allowed me to include each of them openly in this intimate story.

About the Author

Amy Burros graduated from art school in 1973. Two years later she married her high school sweetheart, John Dempsey, after he graduated from college. They have remained in Bergen County, New Jersey, where both were raised. Amy and John adopted their daughter Anne in1985. Leaving her job as a commercial artist immediately, Amy became a "stay-at-home mom."

Anne brought "light" into their lives. She was a four-day-old infant who opened up a new dimension of love to their family. Like most first children she was a born ruler. Almost four years later their second child, Keith, was adopted. He brought "joy" to the family as he always had a unique way of looking for fun in everything he did. Life was sweet.

Five more years down the road, their baby sister was born. After almost nineteen years of marriage, Amy and John gave birth to their third child, Cara. She brought "peace" and a part of the experience they had all missed before. This arrival was just as exciting as the first two were. Cara was a funny chatterbox, who quickly learned how to hold her own with her older siblings.

Amy enjoyed being a full-time wife, mother, nurse-maid, cook, housekeeper and chauffer. She was also an occasional school volunteer and sports fan, who often says, "Parenting is much more complicated than I could have ever imagined. Sometimes, it even gets scary. Still, it is the best thing we ever did!"

At age fifty Amy went back to working outside the home. She took jobs in day care, telemarketing and customer service. All those jobs were adventures and not careers. When the economy changed in 2009 she was let go. Amy reflects, "I could never have imagined then, that only four months later I would be diagnosed with breast cancer and start a journey that would lead to writing a memoir and discover a new passion!"